MW01244141

HONEYBEES, HERBS, AND HEALING

Find your own health in God's natural miracles.

~ FIRST EDITION ~

Alberto Martínez

HONEYBEES, HERBS, AND HEALING

Published by Blue Dragonfly Publishing

www.bluedragonflypublishing.com

ISBN: 9798839659278

DISCLAIMER

This book has been written to introduce the reader to the author's personal experience with natural means of healing such as apitherapy, herbology and naturopathy. The intention is exclusively educational. This book should not be considered a substitute for a licensed physician for your health condition. The author and the publicist discard any legal responsibility for any personal decision of the reader regarding the information contained in this book.

The health recommendations included in this book are based on my training, personal experience, my own research and those of authors in which I believe. Because each person's situation is unique, and because I am not a doctor, I recommend that readers visit a health professional before using the material presented in this book.

Because there is always a risk involved in the consumption or use of anything, and because anyone can be allergic to anything that is in this book or not, please do not use anything if you are not willing to assume your own risk. Consult a doctor or any health professional and seek a second and third opinion for your health condition. The author and publisher do not assume any legal responsibility for the use of the indications suggested in this book.

DEDICATION

A special thanks to Dr. Francisca Romay who taught me that each goal is a new starting point, and always reminded me of the words of José de la Luz y Caballero "Education begins in the cradle and ends in the tomb."

TABLE OF CONTENTS

What You Will Get in This Book

In the following pages the reader will find hundreds of recommendations, many have been scientifically proven, others empirically. I strongly believe in what I recommend but I cannot assure with certainty that what is written here will always work. When it comes to health, there is no single solution that fits everyone.

This book has been written for those who believe in alternative therapies and for those who have no choice but to try something different because what they previously tried did not work for them. This includes what I believe from my own experience and practice and from the experience and practice of others in whom I believe. However, your health is your own responsibility. The decision regarding your health is yours.

The book includes:

- Benefits and proper use of hive products, manufactured and metabolized by bees such as honey, pollen, propolis, royal jelly, wax, bees' bread.
- Products and nutritional formulas.
- Home remedies.
- Western, Chinese and Ayurveda herb remedies.
- Protocols with nutritional supplements such as vitamins, minerals, terrestrial and marine plants, and oils.
- Healing through the use of common foods.
- Suggestions for specific imbalances such as colds, toothache, stomachache, cancer, arthritis, and many more.

If you decide to buy this book, I promise you the following:

- You will have a quick reference to natural remedies for you, your family, and your patients.

- You will find important information that allows you to defend Creationism against the theory of Evolution (evolution exists, but within the same genus, outside the same genus there is no evidence and would deny the theory of chromosomes that is verifiable science)
- You will lose the fear to question and critique modern medicine that believes everything has to be synthetic or scientifically proven by experts in order for it to work.
- You will find solutions for your health condition at a very low cost, sometimes at no cost, that you may find in the yard, in the kitchen, or in the landscape of your own home.

"There are three stages of truth regarding health as well as in other fields of knowledge, which should be fully understood and distinguished from one other: first, something is true but nobody knows it yet; second: something is true and some people know it through experience; and third: something is true and has been verified by scientists"- Henry C Lu

Prologue

The line between reality and fantasy is often blurry. We believe what we want to believe, and we doubt what we want to doubt. Impartiality almost does not exist because we are strongly influenced by the paradigm of our time and our sociocultural environment. Our own thinking is influenced by the thinking and acting of those around us. It has always been like this. In the end, reality usually triumphs, and even becomes truly widespread, but that takes time, sometimes centuries, and requires people willing to think differently and endure the arrogance, prejudice, and mockery of many.

The reality is that although scientific progress is enormous, with regard to the most insignificant animal and plant life, it hides secrets that we do not understand. The word of God tells us in Proverbs 24-13 "Eat, my son, honey, because it is good, and the honeycomb is sweet to your palate." And Matthew 2-11 tells us "And when they entered the house, they saw the child with his mother Mary, and fell down and worshiped him; and opening their treasures, they offered him presents: gold, frankincense and myrrh."

Honey, myrrh and many other herbs are treasures. If the practice proves it irrefutable, then the only thing that limits us to the use of its benefits is the paradigm that blinds us.

With this book, and all my years of study, I hope to help you find natural treatments for your health condition, and to do so with thanks to God for the enormous treasures that nature provides us.

If you decide to follow this book, please do not be afraid to defend its truths. Instead, spread them. Help us to get out of the ignorance imposed upon us in the name of science.

"Health, like freedom, is not a passive object that is delivered or bought but an active process that seeks coherence. It is to sail our own boat in the

sea, without ever reaching port as the final destination. Health is no longer the absence of diseases that freedom is the absence of interference. Both consist of identifying and overcoming obstacles "- Between Paradise and Earth. Harriet Beinfield and Efrem Korngold.

1. Introduction

You've probably once healed some health condition with a tea, soup, or other special meal, or with acupuncture, homeopathy, or some other form of holistic medicine. Has a family member or friend ever been healed of a condition, by natural means, that experts have claimed to be incurable? Have you ever read studies or watched documentaries that spoke of miraculous, inexplicable cases of people or groups that experienced an improvement that modern science (allopathic medicine) doesn't understand?

Your answer to one or more of these questions is most likely "yes".

So, why doesn't that kind of news spread like the wind? Why don't you tell others what you already know is beneficial and economical? Because you are told these anecdotes are not proven in a scientific way, are old-world stories, or that those who told you don't have a degree from a major university.

You fear being ridiculed.

This book will definitely take away that absurd paranoia, and that is an important part of my message.

One thing that all human beings have in common, without exception, is that we are all organic. Therefore, it is irrational that we believe our health has to depend exclusively on inorganic products made in a laboratory, and that we ignore the immensity of natural resources our Creator placed within our reach.

My Personal Story

My love of natural medicine began in 1969 as a beekeeper. Through experimentation and observation, I experienced the benefits of the products of that extraordinary animal that I love so much, the bee.

After coming to the United States in the 80s, and after many jobs in different industries, I decided to get certified as a teach for the state of New Jersey. In studying for my teacher's certification exam, I had to study biology and other sciences. This reignited my love of learning, and of all things natural. From then on, I read books about bees and honey and of other natural remedies. As I taught math in the New Jersey school system, I continued studying natural healing and became certified in various areas of natural medicine.

Back in 2001-2002, I went to a medical doctor for hemorrhoid problems because the pain I had been suffering was finally gone. I told the doctor how I cured it with natural remedies, and I will never forget his reaction. He was furious! He told me that my story is the stuff of tabloid TV programs like Primer Impacto, a Spanish-language TV show that reports outrageous stories such as alien sightings and other pop-culture nonsense.

He referred me to a specialist to take some tests, but I decided not to take them. He insisted that I reconsider, but I already thought about it, and I didn't change my mind. The truth is, the medical doctor didn't believe my story, so how could I trust him if he didn't trust me?

I know that not all medical doctors are like this. I am only narrating my personal experience without adding or removing a single dimension. The benefit of modern medicine is obvious in traumatic cases such as accidents, urgently needed or planned surgeries, cases of heart attacks, difficult births, strokes of the brain and hundreds of other cases.

We cannot deny the altruism of many of its practitioners either, but the sad reality is that a large part of the modern medical system is broken. Today's medical system has an uncontrollable power that undermines individual freedom and corrupts insurances and government health programs. Above all, it is more interested in producing astronomical corporate gains over providing actual health services and benefits to the people.

Because if this, I decided to do my own research. I started taking naturopathy courses and created my own protocols. I decided to study herbology with emphasis and diagnosis based mainly on Chinese medicine, and to read many books and take lots of notes, and to see patients. Among my patients I have seen more-or-less common, easy-to-solve cases, but I have also had complex cases have reinforced my faith in natural medicine and had prompted me to continue practicing and to write this book.

Trust in Natural Medicine

My colleagues from other branches of alternative medicine have noticed that people shy away from talking about natural remedies, even when it has proven positive results for their predicaments.

In one case, I had a patient with cancer who was told that she was terminal and that there was nothing left to do. First, I treated the imbalances she suffered according to Chinese medicine (the branches), then specific herbs for her condition, and now, thank God, she is well. But, when asked, she was reluctant to tell people how she was cured.

In two separate cases I had two patients who could not get pregnant. One of them spent a lot of money on specialists and nothing came of it. Now, after following my treatment, they both have their sons and daughters. One of them did it twice! Yet again, the two women were reluctant to tell people how natural medicine helped them conceive.

To be clear, I don't want to leave the impression that I will always succeed. Of course not. Nothing is certain. The point I'm trying to make is that I couldn't understand why they felt shy or embarrassed about having been successfully treated with natural medicine. I believe they feared being ridiculed for agreeing to a treatment that was not given by a medical doctor or proven by scientific methods. Many educated people make fun of things they don't understand and consider natural medicine a joke, and so my patients feared being thought of as a fool.

My colleagues have had similar experiences, and it is difficult to not take it personally. It can be considered a lack of consideration from the patient, a form of ingratitude, especially because we only have the patient's best interest at heart.

The most amazing example of this phenomena, and one that definitely motivated me to write this book, is provided by Charles Mraz in his book Health and the Honeybee. Charles Mraz was a beekeeper and apitherapist who became famous for using bee sting therapy to treat various ailments. In his book he describes using bee sting therapy to treat a patient, Elijah, suffering from a severe case of arthritis. Elijah had arthritis in almost every joint in his body. He couldn't move. Mr. Mraz applied bee stings every few days, and there were many sessions given the severity of his condition. He was notably better after several treatments.

Elijah moved away a few months later and seven years passed before they met again in New York. A tall, strong man, full of health, approached him and said, "I am Elias, your old neighbor from Middlebury, Vermont." Charles Mraz did not recognize him. When Charles mentioned his treatments with the bee stings, Elias seemed to want to avoid the question as if there was no relationship between the stings and the tremendous physical condition he was in at that time they reunited.

Charles Mraz later learned that this was not an isolated case, that many of his patients refuse to believe that bee stings bring them back to health. Of these cases, Charles Mraz said, "the improvement is 95% bee venom and 5% what they want to believe." *5-p. 25-27. *6-p. 16-28. *7-p. 118-119.

Natural Medicine Deniers

A young man found my website www.NJApitherapy.com from India. He came to the US and made an appointment for his sister's husband. Between him and the patient's brother, Mr. C was carried up to my apartment on the second floor. They carried him because his legs did not move at all. After the first treatment we agreed that I would go to see him at his house, also in New Jersey.

I placed bees on his hands, on his back, along the spine and on acupuncture points B 40 (weizhong), B23 (shenshu), B57 (chenshan), B52 (zhishi), B60 (kunlun), B11 (dashu), St 36 (zusanli). Also along the spine without considering acupuncture points on some visits. He was excited and he didn't care about the number of bees, rather he wanted more. I prepared a food and nutrient recommendation that will be included in the multiple sclerosis protocol later in this book. One day after placing the bees I asked him to get out of bed. He was scared but with my help he stood on my shoulder, for the first time in a long time he held himself up. Multiple sclerosis was decreasing. I was very happy and extremely excited. On the next visit, after 6-8 bites, Mr. C told me to stop, and claimed it wasn't working.

Years later, I am still amazed, because the improvement was evident. I think the reason is explained in the negative influence of others who do not believe in something that is not "scientific." I say this because of Mrs. Maria, a patient who I placed hundreds of bees on in about two years because of her arthritis, the worst of the many I have seen. She assured me that not a week went by without someone telling her that her bee sting treatment was crazy, that it was not recognized by medical science, to which she replied that it was crazy to endure pain without doing anything, and that bees were the only thing that did her good. I include her testimony at the end of the book.

I know that glory must always be given to God, but it is also true that it was God who created bees, herbs, food, and everything else. In medicine, natural treatments are often considered unscientific or inferior. This is why it is not included in medical insurances, and why there is a lack of support and funding for scientific research of natural medicine.

Natural Medicine vs. Modern Medicine

Reason suggests that if in sports you compete on equal terms, why not compete on equal terms in medicine? Why not apply herbs, honey propolis, vitamins, and other natural remedies alongside man-made, manufactured drugs, and observe and compare results?

Instead, the competition is against a placebo. And why is this?

The placebo effect is based on Cartesian theory and is the only method used to verify the effectiveness of a new drug or process. René Descartes said in Rules for Directions of the Mind, Rule IV, "There is need of a method for finding out the truth." So, a method was created to know a drug's true impact on a condition, by comparing it to a placebo. Little relevance is then given to past experiences, unlike other cultures and trends such as Chinese culture and holistic medicine that accept truths from the past and add new truths as they come, including facts that cannot be explained. Cartesian theory, in its eagerness to explain everything, discards a solution that works when its success cannot be explained.

We know that the placebo effect exists in the natural and in the unnatural. Someone takes something perhaps harmless but believes that it does well and is cured by their faith. But it is interesting that many scientists do not accept prayer, supreme form of faith as a method of healing, and base all their research on the placebo effect that is nothing but a subset of faith. Prayer is a superior healing method, of which millions can testify and there are scientific experiments that prove it.

Modern medical science has an aptitude for suspicion, disbelief, and disdain for common experience. Their economic power and their almost absolute mastery of the media and education has allowed them to maintain a propaganda machine that decides what is true and what is not, regardless of the accumulation of empirical knowledge over centuries that has proven their validity.

It is easy to find people who have experienced, either directly themselves or indirectly through someone they know, the benefits of alternative medicine, where it solved ailments that conventional medicine was totally ineffective. Many of us know that it does work, but we refuse to speak of the anecdote as truth so that we may appear scientific before others. We don't want to resist the collective resonance of intellectual slavery, instead we want to follow the majority.

The playing field between Natural Medicine and Modern Medicine is uneven. In sports, the rules are the same for all participants. Whoever wins is congratulated and given medals and awards, no matter how they win. However, in medicine there is no such competition. Something that has resulted in health benefits for thousands of years is neglected because "there is no scientific evidence."

In the Olympic Games in Mexico in 1968, Dick Fosbury was one of the competitors in high jump. His leap was in the form of a half circle with his back to the rod. He was highly criticized for using such a wild technique never before seen by other coaches and sports reporters. He was so different from the others that, even after winning the gold medal, his technique was not only criticized but even banned by some experts. But Dick Fosbury kept winning, his technique kept proving itself successful, and now it is the technique used by almost all competitive high jumpers today.

I apologize to those readers who don't care about sports and competitions at all, but it is very important to highlight the importance of the rules being the same and that happens in sports, chess, golf, car racing, but not in medical science. I would like to see honeybees compete against all those creams for skin problems that are so expensive and often so ineffective. Propolis of bees against antibiotics, the vitamin B complex against nerve tranquilizers, ginger against anti-acids. Competing against a placebo cannot be more scientific than comparing the new against something that many already know is effective.

In my opinion, the economic aspect is the only reason why confrontation on equal terms of the alternative versus the conventional is not allowed. The medical and pharmaceutical industries would lose a lot of money if more natural, and cheaper alternatives proved more effective.

In this book I have included hundreds of different recommendations for your health, but my purpose is not limited to helping you find a possible solution for your health condition. I want to also help you tell others, without the fear that people will believe that you are not "scientific", that you do believe in nature and in all that God has given us for the benefit to our health.

Believing in the "Experts"

Empirical knowledge comes first, everything else comes later, therefore, it should not be a motive of mockery but respect. The truth should be accepted regardless of who formulates it. Unfortunately, this is not the case and that has cost humanity a great price. Those who lead and believe that they are always right have been wrong many times, and their errors have been forgotten. See some of the things that experts claimed as absolute truth:

• The earth is flat. Universities of Europe, including Salamanca

• Television has very few commercial possibilities. Renowned New York Times journalist in 1927, Philo T. Farsworth.

• This "phone" has many problems to be considered a means of communication. Western Union memo, 1876.

Experts also assured that "the heart cannot be operate", "man will never reach the moon", "blood-letting is an effective cure for almost all diseases", "margarine is much healthier than butter", "olive oil is very bad for your health", "wine even in a small amount is harmful to health", "eggs are harmful because they raise cholesterol", "the diet has nothing to do with diseases", "it is better for the health to operate on the tonsils because they are useless", "the appendix should be extracted to improve health because they do not fulfill any function", "a mother's milk is not as nutritious as the infant formulas."

The reader is surely aware of at least several of these statements, some quite recent. Although, as always, when it is known for sure that the wise were wrong, they go on with their wrong theories and you say nothing because you're not a scientist. Most people don't think, they just follow the established rules.

A more recent and constant example is when medical drugs that have been scientifically researched and approved by the FDA, and eventually put on the market, are recalled because of their horrible side-effects or because they are proven ineffective. When this happens, the drug companies simply take the drug off the market and produce a new one in its place. They continue being the "experts" because their drugs are continually reviewed and approved by the FDA. It is a harmful cycle, but because its process is considered scientific it gains the approval of the people over natural medicines.

In my opinion, a drug company's prioritize corporate profit over improving people's health, and all this with the approval of those who are supposed to ensure the health of taxpayers. Every year, without exception, many FDA-approved drugs are removed from the market after they failed to do what was promised, and often because they worsen the condition they were supposed to treat. It is a horrible system, one that cannot be trusted.

True scientists have been ignored throughout history – one great example is Dr. Ignaz Semmelweis (1818-1865). He observed the high mortality rate of women giving birth at the gynecology clinic of the University of Vienna, Austria. Dr. Semmelweis concluded that the main cause was poor hygiene. Doctors and medical students would leave the operating room without washing their hands and then they would tend to women in labor, passing along any infections they may carry. His theory was a matter of mockery. Semmelweis began to receive babies in a clinic outside the university and gave the order that all medical personnel had to wash their hands well. He managed to reduce mortality almost to zero, but even with this proof the critiques continued. Dr. Semmelweis lost his mind, perhaps more worried about his patients than his own luck, and died in a mentally ill center before his 50th birthday.

Many years and thousands of unnecessary deaths later, Dr. Semmelweis's idea was established as a practice by Dr. Joseph Lister (1872-1912). After observing the large number of deaths due to open fractures and very few deaths due to simple fractures, Dr. Lister decided to protect open fractures with carnic acid, thereby achieving excellent results. This principle of antisepsis soon extended to all fields of surgery. Dr. Lister was honored to be the founder of antiseptic surgery, but in an act of generosity, Dr. Lister recognized Dr. Semmelweis as deserving of that honor.

Dr. Barry Marshall, an unknown doctor from a hospital in Perth, Australia, after much research was the first to propose that the stomach ulcer was mainly caused by the H Pylori bacteria. His experiments were unconventional and stress theory was the only truth accepted by the medical community. They mocked him not only in Australia but also in the USA. At a medical conference, a gastroenterologist made a comment that produced laughter in the audience, and in front of his wife who was also part of the conference.

Luckily, Dr. Barry is a man of strong convictions, as it should be, and before rejecting his theory he drank a liquid containing H Pylori and became ill with ulcers. He demonstrated the veracity of his theory and received the 1985 Nobel Prize in Medicine.

The Whole Is More Than the Sum Of Its Parts

"There is an evil which I have seen under the sun, as an error which proceedeth from the ruler: Folly is set in great dignity, and the rich sit in low place." - Ecclesiastes 10: 5-6 (Move this)

I heard on TV the following news: "Recent studies on echinacea herb (angustofolia or purpurea) showed that this herb does not have antibiotic constituents in adequate amounts to provide the effects attributed to it." The echinacea has been used by Native Americans before the arrival of Europeans and is still used in the US and Europe.

Today we know that it is a strong anti-inflammatory, increases the immune system by stimulating T cells, prevents the formation of blood clots and is effective against bacteria and viruses. Here we have one more case in which theory is more appreciated than practice.

Another example, but in reverse, in which a theory is considered more important than practice is the massive distribution of laboratory fluids with which they nourish, or rather, they believe nourish the sick and elderly. In one investigation, laboratory mice were supplied exclusively with one of these nourishing liquids. The capacity to reproduce diminished from one generation to another, all were dying until there was not one left alive. Conclusion: these liquids do not allow procreating and maintaining life in animals that we know can live with almost anything. Despite this, there are more and more laboratory products, not only liquids, and not only for the sick and elderly but also for the general population.

If we make an analogy with sports, we would have to deduce that a person who in his childhood had a stunted growth and did not grow as an adult at a normal height but was short, comparatively weak, of low body and muscle mass could not possibly have a professional career in a sport as demanding as soccer. However, the aforementioned characteristics correspond to those of Lionel Messi, emblematic player of the national team of Argentina, with the highest number of goals scored in a season in the history of the La Liga Spanish League, more goals scored in the history of his club FC Barcelona, and for many the best player in the world.

What should matter most about herbs, honey, food, people, etc., is what they can do, even if the individual components do not correspond to what we understand today, or we think we understand as suitable.

In the organic, the whole is more than the sum of its parts.

I think that food, herbs, propolis, bee venom, etc., are extraordinarily complex mechanisms which contain enormous amounts of information, of which reproduction by man is impossible. Although we can know many characteristics of its components, we cannot explain everything about it. The whole is much more than the sum of the parts that compose it because the whole in natural things is a MECHANISM.

That is the reason why man cannot make an apple even if he knows exactly what all its components are—we cannot arm the mechanism. Something as insignificant as a little board, a nail, a wire, and a hook, it would be said that they are useless, but placed in a special, unique way, it serves to hunt mice. We know how to assemble the mechanism, but any herb, or food contains countless substances, and we simply cannot arm the mechanism. We cannot substitute food created by God with products created in laboratories. Although such products may be food, they will never be real nutrients.

Holistic medicine, or naturopathy, deals with balancing the entire body and this is achieved without always knowing the entire process. The body knows how to do it through its millions and millions of chemical reactions and with the help of the mind. That is not accepted as true science according to the current patterns in which everything has to be systematically deduced, in the Cartesian way.

If a river is diverted for the construction of a dam, and butterflies, bees, birds, frogs, and plants begin to disappear, it is not possible to revert the valley to its previous condition bringing more of what is no longer there because previous living conditions are not present. If the river is brought back to its original channel, there will be a valley that will allow the habitat to return the same as before. As absurd as it may seem, in allopathic medicine the symptoms are given more importance, everything is done thinking about the parts, that's why there are so many "specialists", but few deals with the entire valley.

The placebo effect is also based on Cartesian philosophy and is the only method used to verify the effectiveness of a new drug or process. We know that the placebo effect exists. Someone takes something harmless but believes that it does well and heals.

But it is interesting that scientists who accept the placebo effect do not accept prayer, a supreme form of faith, as a method of healing. Millions can testify to the power of prayer. Experiments have been conducted that demonstrate the effectiveness of prayer even when the patient doesn't know that others are praying for his recovery. Even though prayer is not accepted as a form of healing by science, the placebo effect, a lower form of faith, is.

The placebo effect exists, no one doubts that, but comparing an artificial method or drug with a natural one, knowing in advance that the placebo effect is present in both, seems much better to me if the real objective was to improve or cure diseases.

Holistic medicine too many times tries to explain things based on the Cartesian method and has to change the theory regularly. I think that the natural must be in a different paradigm than the Cartesian. We must accept the truth without trying to show that we know everything, and even more, accepting that perhaps we will never know everything because absolute truth is not always given to men.

Integrating Holistic and Western Medicine

The biggest difference between holistic medicine and Western medicine is that holistic medicine looks for the causes of imbalance and tries to rebalance the body's natural systems, accepting that it cannot know everything that made it possible to achieve that balance, while Western medicine treats symptoms without thinking much about the causes.

Western medicine is far superior to Chinese medicine and other forms of herbology in traumatic cases such as accidents, necessary surgeries (whether urgent or planned in advance), heart attacks, early or normal births, use of drugs for a limited time, strokes, and hundreds of other cases. It also includes the use of modern equipment of extraordinary help in the analysis, diagnosis and treatment of many diseases and imbalances of different types.

An accurate diagnosis by Western medicine can be very useful not only for treatment with such medicine but also for the use of other therapies, such as herbalism, naturopathy, apitherapy, etc.

The use of all modalities of medicine would be the best for the benefit of achieving better health for all at an affordable price within the reach of all budgets. Of course, at the moment it is a chimera, because when there is a belief in the circles of power that a science is the only one, and the rest has no merit. Even when they realize there is nothing left to do, most people still do not give natural remedies a chance.

There are also economic interests to avoid the union of all forms of medicine, I have no doubt about that.

Recently, I heard a senator from the United States exposing his views on health insurance. He never mentioned the advantage that the incorporation of natural products could bring to the treatment of health imbalances and to the pockets of his constituents. Everything he said was to increase funding for allopathic medicine, millions upon millions of tax dollars. Years ago, maybe six, maybe ten, I don't know exactly, that same senator made me feel very optimistic. He said that his brother, who suffered horribly from allergies and who visited the most famous specialists without success, was eventually cured of his allergies with bee pollen. At that time, I thought, "Now we are going to have an unconditional ally in the Senate". How naive I was. Political campaigns are very expensive, and the natural medicine community does not contribute to campaigns, but pharmaceutical companies do, and when they do they are very generous.

The cost of conventional medicine is incredibly high worldwide. The pharmacopoeia that once existed in many countries that included herbs and natural remedies will no longer be found by the reader. I already tried and I think I made a serious attempt. Everything is controlled by the pharmaceutical industries, all but their individual decision to take care of their health and that of their family and friends.

The reader has the right to choose what he thinks is best for him, much of which will be affordable. In this book you will find a huge variety of options, some are in your kitchen, others in the patio, others in the field, in the nearest store, and some can be found online. Many people with limited resources will find solutions to their imbalances, but others with more resources, as happened to the senator's brother, will also be able to relieve themselves with natural things.

I hope with this book to be able to help the millions of people who can no longer deal with the enormous costs of conventional medicine and their side effects. And to those who were assured that there was no solution to their ailment, I offer them a hope and a chance for a cure.

2. Apitherapy

My first encounter with alternative medicine was related to beehive products, as a beekeeper, so we are going to start with apitherapy.

What is Apitherapy?

Apitherapy is the art and science of using hive products for therapeutic purposes, including honey, pollen, royal jelly, bees, wax and bee venom. Bee venom therapy (BVT) involves using live bees, or the injection of bee venom, in order to help people suffering from certain medical conditions that generally do not respond positively to conventional therapies. I use only live bees.

Note: Apitherapy has not been approved by the US Food and Drug Administration, or any other government agency in the USA.

Honey

Honey is the end product of long, tedious work of bees that begins with the location and extraction of the nectar from the flowers and their transportation to the hive. The nectar has a sugar content of between 5% and 60%. The main sugars in the nectar are sucrose, glucose and fructose. Bees add invertase to the nectar. This enzyme converts sucrose into glucose, fructose and maltose while keeping small amounts of sucrose, hydrogen peroxide ($H2O2$) and flavonoids in honey. The viscosity of honeybees is due to the evaporation of water to which bees subject the nectar to convert it into honey. Bees add the very important glucose oxidase enzyme, thereby lowering the Ph (increase the acidity) of honey making it more resistant to fermentation.

The ability to absorb moisture, viscosity, osmotic pressure, low pH, the concentration of sugars and the presence of hydrogen peroxide and flavonoids mean that microbes cannot grow in honey.

The high nutritional power of honey is due in part to its content of vitamins, minerals, enzymes and calorie content of easy absorption and assimilation. It contains vitamin A, beta carotene, all B vitamins, vitamin C, vitamin D, vitamin E, vitamin K, magnesium, sulfur, phosphorus, iron, calcium, chlorine, potassium, iodine, sodium, copper and manganese. *3-p. 48. *7-p. 111-113.

I believe the presence of propolis, royal jelly, wax, and bee venom in honey, although in very small quantities, contribute to the wonderful qualities of honey. They are partly the reason why raw honey, without heating and without super-filtering is therapeutically superior.

Honey is a unique product, a gift from God that has been benefiting humanity since ancient times. Containers containing honey were found in the tombs of the Egyptian pharaohs 4000 years before our era (and was in perfect condition). They were known and consumed by the Assyrians, Greeks, Chinese and Romans. These ancestral cultures believed that daily consumption of honey ensured better health and longevity.

I agree with the ancients, and I am doing very well in terms of my health. I consume honey on a daily basis, and I recommend that if you are not allergic to honey, consume it frequently.

Benefits of Honey

Regular consumption of honey has many benefits. It increases your appetite, increases your salivation, facilitates digestion, increases the immune system, is a light laxative, is anti-anemic, increases athlete's performance, restores low levels of vitamins, minerals, amino acids, and calories.

Two or three tablespoons in the morning could eliminate a stomach ulcer. Eliminates physical fatigue, prevents and helps remove infections in the respiratory system and combats external attack of bacteria in flu cases.

It can be used externally for burns, sores, acne, facial cleansing as well as for skin and eye infections. For the eyes, honey of the Melipona bees (earth bees or sting-less bees) is suggested. I know of a case where a woman diagnosed with glaucoma, with a scheduled surgery, put drops of honey from Melipona bees in her eyes and she no longer needed surgery.

Honey and something else

When combining honey with other substances, it offers great benefits that have been verified by personal testimonies and anecdotes. Some of these combinations have been known for a long time and may have been forgotten, and others have been recently discovered. I have experimented with many of these recommendations, on myself, with family, with friends, and with patients. The results have been excellent.

It's very important to note that the products of the hive, herbs and any substance or nutrient can produce allergy in some people, so it is important to start with a test that contains a minimum dose.

Some combinations include:

- Honey dissolved in a little water helps treat insomnia and calms nerves.

- Heat equal amounts of water and a bit more of lemon juice. Combine the juice and water and dissolve two tablespoons of honey to treat a sore throat.

- Honey dissolved in the juice of a lemon treats colds and diarrhea.

- Two tablespoons of pollen and three tablespoons of honey mixed in a jug of water (five or six glasses of eight ounces or so). Pollen contains more protein than meat and honey and is an excellent nutrient. This mixture can be used:

    o   As a meal substitution to lose weight.

    o   Instead of protein powders.

    o   To increase energy in cases of anemia or chronic fatigue.

    o   To increase sexual potency.

- 1/2 honeybees dissolved in ½ apple cider vinegar can be used to treat knee pain and/or arthritis.

- Place dead bees in a pan over medium heat until they begin to smoke. Remove from the pan and crush them in a mortar until they look like dust. Mix the bee powder with honeybees and apply it on the skin to to treat alopecia (baldness).

- Mix honey with cinnamon for arthritis and/or cancer.

- Peel a leaf of aloe vera (aloe vera) and put everything white in a blender along with six ounces of water and a pound of honeybees. This can be used to treat serious skin problems and digestive problems. You will be amazed at the result.

- Two teaspoons of anise, a teaspoon of ginger powder and a teaspoon of black pepper. Mix everything with honey and form a paste consistency. This is my favorite TRIKATU formula, which is used in Ayurvedic medicine (from India). This is used to treat a cough. ¼ teaspoon or less when the desire to cough comes and every half hour even though at that time you don't have a cough.

- Propolis, marigold (calendula officinalis), neem (azadirachta indica) and plantain (plantago major). Mix everything with honey and apply on skin for any condition, no matter the name of the condition. With this only you paid the price of the book. I have seen really incredible results. One of the substances, propolis is one of the best kept secrets to humanity. It is a pity that something so beneficial to so many imbalances is unknown to most people. In another section I will discuss propolis in depth.

- Honey mixed with natural orange juice can teat gut noises and chronic stomach problems.

- Honey mixed with grapefruit juice can treat stomach ulcers.

Quality Honey

About 90% of products labeled as "pure honey" is actually corn syrup. Current regulations allow you to write "pure honey" on the label even if it is not true. The state of Florida requires a range of pollen in honey so that real honey can be distinguished from fake honey. I hope other states will apply similar measures in the future.

Honey that is heated to high temperature (pasteurization) and then cooled to be easily packaged can be 100% natural but cannot be compared to the one that was never heated and that contains its enzymes without being destroyed by heat. If, in addition, the honey was super-filtered to prevent it from sugaring and with it the particles of wax, pollen, propolis, royal jelly and bee venom were removed, it will no longer have all the therapeutic properties that are known to honeybees.

There are several ways to recognize quality honey that holds real therapeutic properties.

- Natural honey is thick, and sometime it does not have a completely uniform color due to the irregular distribution of pollen, propolis and wax.

- Honey that is sweeten, contrary to popular opinion, is pure honey. This occurs over time in almost all of them, regardless of the floral source, but when the water content is less than 18%, the honey will be sweeten within a week or earlier. In places like the extreme north of the United States, Canada and Ukraine, for example, this honey is consumed without reservation since it is the only one they know, and they also consume the cream-made honey, which is very popular and is very good to spread on bread.

- Pure honey is expensive. Corn syrup is very cheap, but pure honey is not. The handling and packaging of unheated natural honey is much more difficult and the price reflects the extra work.

- You can test the purity of honey by inserting a knife into the honey and letting it drip. The last part should return (like a spring) to the knife and adhere.

- Another way to test the purity of your honey is to add a tablespoon of honey to a glass of water from a height of 1-2 inches. As honey offers a certain resistance to mixing with water, it will stay together at the bottom. If it dissolves before reaching the bottom, then it is not pure honey.

- If you notice that the taste is very sweet but without the taste and consistency that we all know, it could be mixed with corn syrup.

- If the color is too light, too dark, or too uniform, this could be an indication that it is not pure honey.

"You should not be ashamed to ask an ordinary person if something would be useful to you as a remedy, because I think that the art of medicine as a whole was discovered that way" - Hippocrates

Bee Pollen

Pollen is the male seed of flowers. It cannot be a uniform product because it depends on the flowers that the bees have visited, which is also the reason their color varies from a very intense yellow to a fairly dark gray.

Pollen is rich in vitamins B1, B2, B5 (pantothenic acid), B6 and B12, it also contains vitamins A, C, E, folic acid and carotenoids as well as amino acids and proteins (20%). It contains routin and HGH (Human Growth Hormone) and minerals such as calcium, copper, iron, magnesium, phosphorus and more. Pollen is digested very easily and is not considered an herb or a vitamin but a food that has the most essential nutrients to preserve life.

Pollen has been used in cases of allergies, anemia, appetite regulator, asthma, chronic fatigue, low immune system, impotence, infertility, ulcers, prostate problems, menopause, kidney problems, weight control, high blood pressure and to improve performance in sports. *1-p. 16-20. *3-p. 19-29. *4-p. 35-37. *7-p. 21-32.

Most recent scientific research on pollen has originated in Europe. Unfortunately, the scientific community in the United States has shown very little interest in such investigations, much less in the undeniable historical truth that pollen, due to its nutritional characteristics and its ability to replace a meal when the need was pressing, has been used since times ancient by the Roman Legions, the ancient Greeks and by the troops of Charlemagne.

"Where everyone thinks alike, no one thinks very much" - Walter Lippman 1889-1974

Bee Propolis

Propolis is a resinous substance collected by bees, mixed with wax and partially metabolized by the action of enzymes produced by bees. Propolis contains all vitamins with the exception of vitamin K. It contains 13 of the 14 minerals that the body requires, minus sulfur. Propolis varies in color and composition from one sample to another, but generally they are all rich in the following substances: Vitamin A (carotene), Vitamin B complex, such as B1, B2, B3 and a mixture of Bioflavonoids. It contains Biotin, Calcium, Magnesium, Iron, Zinc, Potassium, Phosphorus, Manganese, Cobalt and Copper, and like all other products in the hive, it also has unidentified substances. Propolis has antibacterial, antiviral, antibiotic, anti-fungal, anti-inflammatory and antioxidant characteristics.

Propolis has been used to protect the body from imbalances such as allergies, herpes, throat problems, nasal congestion, respiratory problems, flu, colds, colds, wounds, ulcers, acne, burns, cancer, dental care (some good pastes contain propolis), skin problems, liver protection, anemia.

My belief of propolis is very firm. Long ago, I found a mouse killed by bees in one of my hives, and it was covered with propolis. I got him out of there and I could tell he didn't smell like anything at all. If you've ever found a dead mouse, you know they rot quickly and smell horrible. The rotten odor is hard to bear, but the antibacterial and anti-fungal properties of propolis kept the mouse from rotting. My experience is not unique, other beekeepers have had the same. It's not wonder why propolis was used by ancient cultures to mummify corpses.

Hundreds of scientific studies around the world have demonstrated the extraordinary properties of propolis, and the hive itself is the best example. Bees apply propolis to the hive and thereby protect themselves from everything that inevitably can invade their residence: bacteria, fungi, microbes, etc. Such a high level of protection cannot be achieved in hospitals and clinics no matter how often they are cleaned and sterilized.

A theory regarding the ability of the propolis to eliminate viruses suggests that the propolis covers the protein layer of the virus and does not allow it to reproduce. Eventually, the body eliminates it. *1-p. 8-9,20-21,107-119. *3-p. 19-23. *7- pg. 1116-118.

"In theory, there is no difference between theory and practice, but in practice there is." - Yogi Berra.

Royal Jelly

Royal jelly is a secretion fully synthesized by the hypo-pharynx and the jaw gland of worker bees between 5 and 10 days old.

This is the only nutrient given to queen bee cells and almost the only food the queen bee consumes. The queen bee weighs 200 mg and measures 17 mm compared to 125 mg and 12 mm of the worker bee. The queen bee lays between 2000 and 2400 eggs a day, weighing 200 times its own weight, and contains a large number of different vitamins, 20 amino acids, DNA, RNA, gelatin, a collagen precursor, hormones and unknown substances that have never been isolated in laboratories.

This extraordinary substance can help correct more imbalances than any other substance on earth. The list includes: menopause, impotence, infertility, hormonal imbalance, endocrine system disorders, viral infections, bacterial infections, low immunity, skin wrinkles, skin tags, chronic fatigue, heart problems, high cholesterol, high blood pressure, control of weight, retarded growth, eczema, ulcers, mononucleosis, anabolic support (athletic ability), diabetes, depression, arthritis, lack of memory, cancer, liver problems, Parkinson's disease, anemia and spleen infections.

Royal jelly has been used as a nutritional supplement to benefit the immune, cardiovascular, endocrine, and nervous systems.

It may seem like royal jelly covers a lot, but consider this: the queen bee can live 5 years while the worker bee lives 6 weeks and both come from the same type of egg, with the only difference being the queen bees consumes royal jelly exclusively. *1-p. 23-24, 165-166. *3-p. 7-16. *4-p. 52-58. *7-p. 114-115.

"To be absolutely certain about something, one must know everything or nothing about it." - Olin Miller.

Beeswax

Beeswax is an impermeable substance composed of the mixture of around 300 components, the most abundant of which does not exceed 8% of the total. Therefore, its complexity is such that it is impossible to synthesize or duplicate. One curious fact is the composition of the wax is extraordinarily uniform regardless of the species of bee that produces it.

Wax cannot be digested by mammals (including humans). Some think that consuming it internally can help in certain imbalances, not only because of its high content of vitamin A but because of the effect it produces in the body that, although not can be demonstrated in the scientific way imposed, it could be true.

I believe that honey that has not been super filtered and therefore contains suspended wax particles is still superior, and when I see a little bit of wax in the honey that I consume I simply swallow it along with the honey. In Ecuador there is a therapy, I clarify that anecdotal, which suggests making very tiny balls of wax and swallowing them in order to treat broken bones that won't heal. I have not had any experience with that therapy, but if I had a broken bone that does not heal, I would not hesitate to try to see what happens.

Chewing wax can help eliminate or reduce tartar from the teeth and strengthen the gums. Honey in honeycomb has been recommended to combat asthma since ancient times and honey in honeycomb is nothing other than honey and wax, therefore, wax plays an important role in this therapy.

Beeswax is used in cosmetics. In fact, you can't talk about cosmetology without considering wax. Beeswax is excellent for the skin.

Soaps that contain beeswax are of high quality, in my personal opinion, and are the best soaps out there. If you suffer from unexplained itching, without having anything on your skin, it is very possible that the problem lies in the toxic and allergenic substances included in the manufacture of commercial soaps. Beauty creams, lip crayons, crayons for cracks of the lips, skin masks, creams to remove chicken legs on the face, etc., contains beeswax.

The medicinal use of beeswax includes aromatherapy where it is used in ointments as a base and in formulas in combination with herbs, essential oils and other substances. Beeswax candles alone are a form of aromatherapy, they burn slowly, produce a relaxing flame and their smell calms and gives us a sense of peace that makes us feel very good.

Ear Cone Candling

Ear cone candling is a painless therapeutic procedure consisting in connecting a wax made cone to the ear. The cone is lit and a vacuum is formed. Because of the differences in pressure created, the excess wax and debris is removed. At the same time, the vacuum stimulates blood and lymph circulation. In my experience, the recipient generally feels lightheaded. Ear cone candling can help relieve chronic ear infections in children and adults, alleviates the head and upper respiratory area and it is a tonic for stress reduction. Ear cone candling is almost unknown today but ancient Egyptians, Chinese, Tibetans and Greeks used this method for centuries.

I learned about this therapy and how to use it through Annie Van Alten, from Carlisle, Ontario, Canada, a true expert with years of experience in this technique and in apitherapy in general. She was one of the speakers at a convention I attended in North Carolina, sponsored by the American Apitherapy Society of which I am an apitherapist and beekeeper. *1-p. 8-24. *4-p. 186-187.

"It is a silly young scientist who does not soon learn that the Court of the Inquisition is still sitting judging what is not orthodox. In 1616, Galileo was forced to submit to the orthodoxy of the theologians of the time. We have an equivalent Court today in a network of bureaucratic and political rules. All well intentioned, but its cumulative effect manages to exert a powerful pressure on the orthodox. Our brilliant young people need to be allowed a little more freedom and the opportunity to prove themselves as original thinkers, without being hampered by the system towards the traditional, sometimes through unimaginative channels." - W. Grierson.

Bee Venom

Someday (I will almost certainly not be present to enjoy it), two eminent researchers of bee venom therapy – Bodog F Beck, MD and Charles Mraz – will receive the honor and respect that they amply deserve. Bodog F Beck published "The Bible of Bee Venom Therapy" in 1935 and Charles Mraz published "Health and The Honeybee" in 1995, both left an extraordinary legacy to all of us who practice this therapeutic modality, and to all of humanity. Their detractors will be on the same level as those who assured Christopher Columbus that the Earth is flat.

Bee venom therapy, BVT, involves placing live bees or injecting bee venom in order to help people suffering from certain medical conditions that generally do not respond positively to conventional therapies. I use only live bees.

Note: Apitherapy has not been approved by the US Food and Drug Administration, or any other government agency in the USA.

What can be treated with bee venom?

Some of the most common problems include: Arthritis, Asthma, Bursitis, Bronchitis, Cancer, Corns, Cysts, Eczema, Herpes, Irregular Periods, Low Back Pain, Lupus, Multiple Sclerosis, Myalgia (Muscle Aches), Menstrual Cramps, Neuralgia , Psoriasis, Sciatica, Pain in the elbows (tennis elbow), Varicose Veins, Lou Gehrig's disease and others. Someone said: "If everything has failed, treat the bee sting" *1-p. 213-220,222-224. *4-p. 73-81. *5-p. 46-47.36-38, 22-24, 61.66. *6-p. 169-187.

Note: This list does not guarantee that all these conditions are always cured with BVT bee venom, in addition, this list does not include all the ailments that can be treated with bee venom therapy.

What happens if I am allergic to bee venom?

Contrary to popular belief, bee venom allergy is very rare, only 7 of a thousand people statistically show allergies. Of this proportion, only a small percentage show serious risks (anaphylactic shock), which should be treated with Epinephrine (EpiPen) and Benadryl. In any case, your health is my priority, therefore ALL treatments are preceded by an allergy test.

The first test should consist of a single bite. In the next sessions, the number of bites can be increased and ice can be placed beforehand in the area where the bee is to be placed, which greatly reduces pain without affecting the therapeutic result.

Curiosities of the bees

The wonderful practical knowledge of bee chemistry can be found in the manufacture of honey, wax, propolis and bees bread that bees produce by adding enzymes, different according to what they manufacture. They also know about communication since the exploratory bees communicate to the other bees where the nectar sources are found through a dance, and these can go on their own, without being guided, to these nectar sources.

In mathematics, bees are a natural wonder. We have known for some time that the honeycomb has the perfect figure to store the largest volume and at the same time the greatest possible weight without breaking. For that, knowledge of limit theory and calculus is required, or to have achieved it through trial-error, as evolutionary theory suggests, although there is no evidence in paleontology of honeycombs different than the current ones. The third theory states that they were programmed so that they knew how to do it from the beginning of their existence. You decide, but the math is present.

But there is more. Scientists have discovered that bees fly the shortest possible route between the flowers they visit, thereby solving the postman's problem. Dr. Nigel Raine from the Royal Holloway School of Biological Science and his team used powerful computers and artificial flowers to investigate whether bees follow their route based on the order in which they saw the flowers or if they guided the shortest distance. They discovered that once bees explore the location of the flowers, they fly the shortest distance to visit them.

All the possible ways in visiting a set of flowers is determined by what is known as permutations. If you visit three flowers, say A, B, and C, the possible ways are: A-B-C, A-C-B, B-A-C, B-C-A, C-A-B, C-B-A. You have a total of six possible ways to visit three flowers. In mathematical terms, to find all the different possible permutations of a set of flowers, you use the factorial formula, denoted by the "!" symbol.

For example,

If you visit 3 flowers: $3! = 3 \times 2 \times 1 = 6$

If you visit 5 flowers: $5! = 5 \times 4 \times 3 \times 2 \times 1 = 120$

If you visit 10 flowers: $10! = 10 \times 9 \times 8 \times 7 \times 6 \times 5 \times 4 \times 3 \times 2 \times 1 = 3,628,800$

And if they visit a few more, the number of permutations is so large that the numbers do not fit in a line of computers. How do bees do it?

3. Common Herbs and Home Remedies

"Then God said, 'I give you every seed-bearing plant on the face of the whole earth and every tree that has fruit with seed in it. They will be yours for food. And to all the beasts of the earth and all the birds in the sky and all the creatures that move along the ground – everything that has the breath of life in it – I give every green plant for food.' And it was so."-Genesis 1: 29, 30

The use of plants as a means of fighting diseases was the first form of medicine. Traditional Chinese medicine, for example, began more than 3000 years ago, and began with herbology. Other modalities of this medicine such as acupuncture, tuina (Chinese massage), qi gong (breathing exercises and gentle movements) and tai chi were incorporated much later.

Traditional Chinese medicine is based primarily on a book written many years before Christ. The Huangdi Neijing, also titled The Yellow Emperor's Classic of Medicine, is an ancient text on health and disease said to have been written by the famous Chinese emperor Huangdi around 2600 BC.

That book was a classic then, and continues to be a classic today, because in traditional Chinese medicine, and in herbalism in general, the truths are still valid, contrary to Western medicine in which what they prescribe today will be obsolete within one or two decades. Books recommended today in medical schools will have no value in a short time because everything changes continuously in a type of medicine in which what determines the truth is "the law of the negation of the negation" and in which "the new denies the old". Cartesian concepts are widely used in Marxist societies, such as Cuba and the former socialist countries, but also in non-Marxist societies of the West.

In the next few sections you will find natural remedies and herbs found in traditional Chinese medicine that are used to treat common ailments. Everything will not be effective every time in all people, but many times it will be. Remember that as with drugs, we can also be allergic to any herb or food, so I recommend you start with minimal amounts and be careful to prevent possible allergic reactions.

Aloe Vera

(aloe vera) Other names: lu hui (pinyin), kumai (Sankrit), sabila (Spanish)

Aloe Vera is one of the plants in the Bible and is one of the few plants that appeared in all pharmacopoeias because of its undeniable benefits, it is no longer the case, because now nothing natural is considered medicine by those who have the political and economic power in the world. But it is good to clarify to all that perhaps the only thing that all people have in common is that we are ORGANIC, and on the organic we depend to sustain our lives, and pretend that everything that serves as medicine has to be INORGANIC, is the height of arrogance and folly, and I say more, stupidity.

Aloe Vera is native to the Mediterranean region, is found throughout the Caribbean and in Continental America, its cultivation has been expanded to other regions and almost everywhere in the world can be obtained due to modern means of communication and transportation.

Part used: The gelatinous part, the green is discarded.

The first use of aloe in Cuba was to cure and prevent the distemper of chickens, throwing a piece of a leaf cut in the water that was given to chickens. I have testimonies of the effectiveness of this use.

Asenjo, CT, wrote in Notes on the Medicinal Plants of Puerto Rico, Journal of Agriculture, Puerto Rico in June 1937.

"Aloe vera is a tonic for the liver and spleen, excellent for the female reproductive system. The powder is a powerful laxative, so whoever uses it should do it in small doses."

I have recommended and successfully treated aloe vera against stomach and skin problems prepared as follows: Jelly is separated from green, careful to discard all green. You put all the gelatin in the blender, add 8 ounces of water +/- and a pound of raw honey (not heated, did not know filtered, not radiated), and shake. The dose depends on the condition, one to three tablespoons a day is sufficient in most cases. It is effective in cases of constipation (constipation), any skin condition that is related to the digestive system, (most according to TCM and modern western herbology), glandular inflammation, obesity, hepatitis, fatty or elongated liver, imbalances of the spleen, herpes, tumors, to counteract the effects of radiation or chemotherapy, menopause, bursitis, psoriasis, hemorrhoids, and in external use in cases of minor accidental burns, cuts and skin conditions.

*10-p. 819-821. *11-p. 33-37.

Anamú

(Petiveria alliacea) Other names: namu (Cuba), mapurite (Venezuela), hierba de las gallinitas, zorrillo (México), apasote (Guatemala), Ipacina (Nicaragua), Pipi (Argentina), guinea hen weed (Jamaica).

The anamú has been used against toothaches, fevers, rheumatism, paralysis, venereal diseases, scorpion stings, psoriasis, asthma, hysteria, and other nervous diseases. In recent times it has been used in cancer cases and in cancer prevention. Its flavor is extraordinarily unpleasant if it is prepared in the form of tea. You can put several leaves in a jug of water, wait for the next day and so it can be taken without it being a great sacrifice. Another option is to consume the anamú in capsules.

Pregnant women should not use this herb.

In Sinaloa, Mexico, the leaves are used to be tied to the forehead or placed in hats to relieve the headache.

*9-p. 158-163.

Angel's Trumpet

(Datura arborea) (Brugmansia arborea) Other names: bijarra, flor de campana (Cuba), cornucopia, campana de Paris (Puerto Rico), floripondio (Colombia, Perú, Ecuador, México)

In Mexico, studies were conducted on this plant at the National Medical Institute of Mexico, when medical institutions still included medicinal plants as part of the pharmacopoeia. They found no interesting benefits in it. The reason I include the bell is to warn that it is not used at all, because the bell is narcotic and poisonous. It does not always kill, but it can decrease the cognitive ability of those who use it as a drug, as a substitute for marijuana, for example. The benefits attributed to it are not included because there are many non-toxic herbs that give better results. The bell is an ornamental plant, and nothing more.

*18-p. 33-34, 37, 109.

Apple Vinegar

Many people suffer from gastric reflux and have made them believe that they suffer from excess acid in the stomach, so they recommend antacids, of course they never take away the problem but they get worse. Antacids and antibiotics alkalize the stomach and thereby make the pathogenic bacteria multiply and the good ones decrease, mushrooms proliferate and the lack of energy increases due to the decrease in food assimilation and the affectation of production and absorption of vitamin B12. Two or three tablespoons of organic apple cider vinegar per day may be the solution.

Apple cider vinegar is also very effective in combating skin fungus, those that itch within the ears, those of the sexual organs and close to them and those that come out on the elbows. It could also be useful in foot fungus.

Artemisia

(Artemisia vulgaris) Other names: mugwort, sagebrush, wormwood (English), ai ye (pinyin, Chino)

The cooking of artemisia can be used in cases of delayed menstruation, dislikes, frights, poor blood circulation, in cases of epilepsy and to expel worms.

It is interesting that the use of this herb has some common uses in western herbalism and traditional Chinese medicine where, according to Dan Benski and Andrew Gamble, it heats the womb and calms the fetus, reduces abdominal pain, and could help in cases of infertility or "cold uterus".

Artemisia is the only herb used in the manufacture of "moxa", which is like a tobacco that is used in traditional Chinese medicine to give heat and with it stimulate acupuncture points. This technique is very effective and will be explained at the end of the book for those who want to deepen and delve into the field of traditional Chinese medicine.

*9-p. 178-181. *13-p. 259-260.

Aspirin

In cases of calluses, an aspirin is sprayed and placed in the callus with a band-aid. It can aid in removing the callus.

Avocado

(Persea Americana)

Place small leaves and branches in boiling water to combat excess uric acid (T. Peckolt).

Most medicines in the 1940s were based on the leaves and branches of the avocado when uric acid is involved, according to Juan Tomas Roig in Aromatic or Poisonous Plants of Cuba, first edition, 1945.

The fruit of the avocado is an excellent source of vegetable oil, it is rich in vitamins, proteins, minerals, calories, antioxidants, protects the health of the eyes, is good for the hair and excellent for the protection of the skin. It is said to help lower cholesterol thanks to the presence of oleic acid.

I believe that if avocado helps lower cholesterol, it is not only because of a single ingredient. It is my opinion that nutrients are MECHANISMS, determined by an extraordinarily large amount of INFORMATION, impossible for man to decipher.

There are more than 500 varieties of avocados. The highest per capita consumption of avocados is in Mexico, a country that does not conceive of life without avocado. I believe that Mexicans are exempt from so many ailments due to avocado being and important part of their everyday diet.

Bamboo

(Bambusa vulgaris)

The use of bamboo for medicinal purposes was very limited in Cuba even in the middle of the last century, when medicinal plants were much better known and appreciated than in later times. The reason that it has been included is due to the use that is given to it in Chinese medicine, very important as I think, and because this plant is present throughout the continent, within the reach of anyone who decides to treat it.

The leaves and soft part of the plant have the botanical name bambusa breviflora, Zhu Li in Pinyin. It is used for cough, paralysis of the hands or feet, hemiplegia and dizziness. In case of stroke, a strong tea along with ginger is recommended.

The solid inside part of the bamboo has the botanical name caulis bambusae, Zhu Ru in Pinyin. To use it, you have to cut and crack the cane and remove the fiber from the inside out. The outer part is discarded. This cooking requires a lot of time to extract nutrients. It is used to stop vomiting, stop bleeding, to stop bleeding from the nose and to stop vomiting with blood. If supplied with ginger the effect is even better.

Studies showed that this herb can be stored for a long time in a closed container without diminishing its properties.

*13-p. 182-183. *9-p. 279-280.

Bermuda Grass

(cynoden dactylon) (capriola dactylon) (cynoden dactylon) (panicum dactylon) Other names: grama, grama de Bermuda, pasto Bermuda, yerba Bermuda, yerba del prado, yerba fina (Spanish) capin de cidade (Brasil)

The grass has been studied at the University of Allahabad, in India, where they discovered its properties for the treatment of urinary tract infections, prostatitis, syphilis and dysentery.

They also studied their glycemic potential in a study with mice and found that rats treated with extracts of this plant lowered blood sugar levels by almost 50% when the appropriate dose was supplied. It was concluded in the study that grass could be an alternative medication to fight diabetes. This plant is commonly used in India where it has these names in different languages spoken there: Sankrit: bhargavi, doorwa, granthi, sveta.

Hindi: doorva, doob. Tamil: arugo, aruvam-pillu, mooyar-pul. Bengali: Durba.

Kannada: karuka-pullu. Marathi: doorba, hariali. Punjabi: dub, kabbar, size.

Telugu: garika, gerike, haryali.

The rhizomes of this plant were known in the 1940s in pharmaceutical terms as Grama Mayor, and was then an official drug used WORLDWIDE. F Cainas in his book Cuban Medicinal Plantsp. 175 says "The root is used successfully as a purifying, diuretic, expectorant and febrifuge, if the decoction or maceration is drunk three or four times a day." Today we know the high chlorophyll content of this and other grasses such as chicken leg and horse and guaratero grass (Venezuela), and yerba de guinea (Cuba). It is curious that this herb, subject to jokes and contempt for the last 50 years, is gradually gaining recognition from many. In New York City, near the famous Madison Square Garden I saw two establishments where they prepare grass juice harvested in trays where they cut the grass with scissors and prepare the juice (they add water, as should be done with all juices very rich in chlorophyll).

Bitter Grass

(Paspalum conjugatum)

This herb is spread throughout the Caribbean, southern United States and Continental America. In Argentina there are two species of similar properties, paspalum notatum and the paspalum vaginatum that is known there as "gramilla". In the book titled Medicina Vegetal Plantas Medicinais by Vicente J Morra, the author explains that roots are endowed with diuretic, purifying, refreshing and anti-inflammatory properties, and are administered in cases of liver, kidneys and urinary tract diseases as well as in cases of gastritis, colds and to combat fever and blood pressure.

Argentina is one of the countries who has its own pharmacopoeia that included herbs and natural remedies. I heard about the grass on many occasions in my youth, but at that time I was not interested in herbalism and did not pay attention to the details of the benefits of this plant, but I remember that it was very esteemed and I never heard it be harmful to anyone.

Bitter Melon

(Momordica charantia) Other names: cundeamore (Spanish), wild balsam apple (English), melao de San Caetano (Brasil)

The used parts of this plant, much visited by the hummingbird are the leaves, the fruit and the seeds, although some practitioners consider that it is preferable not to use the seeds.

Cundeamor has a bitter taste that we are not accustomed to in Latin America, however, in the Philippines there is a high consumption of cundeamor in salads. The therapeutic properties attributed to this plant include: Liver imbalances, colitis, is used to lower blood sugar levels in both Ayurveda (Indian) medicine and traditional Chinese medicine. It is recommended in all types of cancers, skin ulcers, anemia and bronchitis. Dr. Juan Tomas Roig said that this was one of the plants with more applications in popular medicine in Cuba, and attributed vermicidal properties to the cundeamor, and according to Teodoro Pekhol "it is an emmenagogue, it establishes the menstrual flow of women."

In the Dominican Republic, cundeamor is produced to export to the communities of Hindus and Chinese residents in the United States, but it also exists in the fields, wild, and even in the yards of many houses throughout the Caribbean and in Continental America from the United States to Argentina. Don't be shy, try it and spread the news of it's success in your treatment, which is highly possible. *9-p. 355-356.

Blessed Thistle

(Cnicus benedictus) Other names: Cardo Bendito (España), Cardo Santo (Portugal), Chardon Benit (Francia)

This somewhat unpleasant herb with a bitter taste is native to Europe and naturalized in North America, but it grows well in tropical climates. Its properties coincide with those of Milk Thistle (silybum marianun), an herb of the Bible that is considered one of the best, if not the best, herbs for cleaning the liver of toxins. It has been used since the last century to stimulate appetite, improve digestion, imbalances of the urinary system, constipation and ulcers. Today it is recommended in cases of cirrhosis, and hepatitis.

*11-p. 163-166. *9-p. 294-297.

Burweed

(Xanthium chinense) (xanthium strumarium) Other names: guizazo, guizazo de Baracoa (Cuba); bardana (Puerto Rico); burdock (English); Can Er Zi, Niu Bang Zi (pinyin)

The genus xanthium includes 25 species, all native to the Americas but propagated and used medicinally in Europe, Asia and America. Gómez de La Maza in his book Flora Habanerap. 573 says that "it was used to treat goiter, herpes, cancer and to dye hair blonde." This plant was included in the list of plants tested as anticancer by the National Cancer Institute in Maryland, United States. It is currently used in western herbalism, Ayurveda and traditional Chinese medicine.

Uses: TCM. Niu bang zi is used as a diuretic, blood purifier in cases of rheumatism, gout, cystitis, chronic skin conditions including acne and psoriasis. In Ayurveda it is recommended in cases of itching, scratching, inflammation of the skin, toxins in the blood, deficiencies of the lymphatic system, inflammation of the kidneys and high blood pressure. In western herbalism it is used in cases of breast imbalances in women, possibly because it cleanses the lymphatic system. Also in skin conditions, including acne and psoriasis as it is a strong blood cleanser, and in liver conditions.

*9-p. 495-496. *13-p. 162-163. *20- page 1114-115.

Cabbage Juice

For foot fungus, internally and externally, acidity (cabbage is highly alkaline), stomach aches, stomach ulcers.

Carob Tree

(Albizia lebbeck) (acacia lebbeck) (monosa lebbeck)

Tea is made with the seed using only half in three cups of water and this is a very effective remedy against diarrhea.

One cup per day might be enough, but if the diarrhea ceases it is advisable to stop taking it because if it continues it is possible to stop defecating for the next two or three days.

Cedar

(Mexican Cedrela)

The bark and resin were used in Cuba and in Mexico for the treatment of fever and epilepsy. Baking with the leaves for toothache. The cooking of the leaves and the bark together was mixed with burning water or alcohol to make a liniment in friction against pain produced as a result of blows or falls.

Chamomile

(matricaria chamomilla) Other names: manzanilla (Spanish)

Chamomile was introduced in Cuba in 1939, but it was already known since before it was imported from Spain. Over time, chamomile became the most popular medicinal herb in Cuba because it could be grown anywhere, without any setback, in any type of terrain.

Chamomile helps fight chronic insomnia with 3-4 cups per day. I recommended this to a friend who had insomnia for many years and it soon went away.

It is also effective in cases of irritability, nervousness, unnecessary aggressiveness, stomach problems such as gas, indigestion, stomach pain, stomach inflammation. Chamomile is effective in cases of skin imbalances, taken in the form of tea or in external use of the same tea.

Chamomile has natural antibacterial properties. Cotton balls soaked with warm, not hot, Chamomile tea can be very effective in eliminating discomfort in the eyes which are often caused by pathogens.

*10-p. 614-619. *12-p. 119-120, 129, 133, 136, 139-140, 152, 154, 156, 158, 171, 176, 198, 201, 204, 215-216, 218, 222, 226, 233, 241.

Cinnamon

(Cinnamomum cassia)

Cinnamon helps to raise blood pressure, and achieves it quickly. It has been used in cases of indigestion, diarrhea, fungi, and viruses. It helps metabolize blood sugar, so it could help in cases of diabetes. It is used in cases of rheumatism, tuberculosis, bronchitis, herpes, menstrual problems, and prevents gum problems. It also helps with cold in arms and legs, impotence, frequent urination, weak back and lack of appetite.

*13-p. 301-303. *18-p. 20, 33,36-37, 75,220. *9-p. 287-288.

Coconut Tree

(Cocos nucifera)

Coconut water is an excellent coolant and a very good diuretic, I think that as much as cranberry, but it tastes much more pleasant than cranberry. The tender coconut is a moderate laxative; the roots were used last century against diarrhea and dysentery. The shell is very astringent (reduces secretions, firm tissues and organs, reduces inflammation and hemorrhoids). Milk eliminates the swelling of the breasts of women who breastfeed children.

Coconut oil is the best of nature, contrary to what people have been saying for the past 30 years. The benefits of coconut oil include: heart protector, strengthens the immune system, promotes weight loss, increases the absorption of nutrients and minerals, fights bacteria and viruses, is used to combat herpes, is excellent for skin and hair (also spread on the hair), against cancer and diabetes, bladder infections, gum problems, and much more. Coconut oil is perhaps the best for frying because it is very stable, little vulnerable to oxidation. In the section of neuropathy we will include more information about this wonder of nature, coconut oil.

*16-p. 2-177. *17-p. 13-66. *9-p. 320-322.

Cold water

It is recommended in cases of burns, hemorrhages, bumps (remember not to eat anything for several hours after the bump), fever, exhaustion, hypertension, insomnia, and to strengthen the body even if you are not sick. It is obvious that if it involves severe burns or affecting a large part of the body surface, urgent medical assistance is the best option. Here we refer to the steam from the pressure cooker, the electric iron that we accidentally touch, a little oil that jumped out of the pan, etc. First aid can be entrusted to cold water until we receive professional help if it is necessary.

Cold water baths can help fight digestive imbalances, insomnia, and lack of energy.

Corn

(zea mays) Other names: yu mi xu (pinyin)

Corn silk constitute an official drug that was listed in all pharmacopoeias. It is used in diseases of the urinary tract due to its diuretic action. The silk or hairs of corn was used as a diuretic in the fields of Cuba in the 1930s through the 1940s. In Chinese medicine it is used very frequently. I highly recommend it in cases of urinary system conditions. Corn silk benefits the gallbladder. Recently it has been recommended in cases of high blood pressure.

*10-p. 583-585. *13-p. 150-151.

Dandelion

(Taraxacum officinale)

This plant, originally from Europe, is highly appreciated by beekeepers in the United States because it is very melliferous. The therapeutic properties attributed to this plant include: cancer, diabetes, skin problems, liver toxin cleanser, hepatitis (specific), ulcers, edema, cleanses the lymphatic system, gallbladder imbalances, tumors. The dandelion leaf is excellent as a salad.

Eucalyptus

(Eucalyptus maculata)

Several eucalyptus leaves are placed in a bowl of water and put on the fire. When it starts to boil, breathe the steam while holding a towel held with both hands over your head so that less steam escapes. This remedy is recommended in cases of nasal congestion, and respiratory problems. If you add laurel the effect may be even greater.

Cainas in his book Medicinal Plants of Cuba,p. 76 tells us "decoction of resin eucalyptus is effective in the cure of diabetes, asthma, influenza, tuberculosis and angina pectoris."

"The leaves of all eucalyptus are astringent, febrifuge and antiseptic. They are rich in tannin and contain an essential oil that is used topically for the cure of sores, ulcers and other diseases of skin tissues. In infusion and pectoral pastes to fight colds and diseases of the respiratory tract and digestive tract; being also used its leaves with the most flattering success in the attacks of diabetes."- Juan Tomas Roig.

Interesting is the accumulation of knowledge and the similarity of uses of eucalyptus in herbalism of the first third of the last century and modern herbalism, everything is almost the same. We must also note the "obscurantism" to which in the name of "science" we have been subjected for so long. I want to reiterate my personal opinion that there is nothing that does not have a cure and there is nothing that cures something every time for all people. For that reason it is essential to have a wide range of options that allow everyone to have the opportunity to find the solution to our health condition.

*9-p. 411-415. *19-p. 185, 239, 247, 272,299-302.

Fennel

(Foeniculum vulgare) Other names: hinojo dulce (España), finocchio (Italia), aneth fenoil (Francia), shatapushpa (Sankrit), xiao hue xiang (pinyin)

Fennel is used in cases of indigestion, stomach gas, difficulty or burning when urinating, stomach pains, childhood cramps and to increase breast milk in women who breastfeed. It is available in capsules.

Flax, Flaxseed, Flax Seeds

(Linum usitatissimum)

One tablespoon is enough to fight constipation (constipation), helps prevent strokes, and could help in cases of chronic problems such as psoriasis and arthritis. It can help prevent arteriosclerosis, helps prevent blood clots, and according to recent studies, helps lower homocysteine levels in the blood. It is perhaps the richest nutrient in omega-3 from plant sources, which is why it is considered a protector of the heart. Just add a tablespoon of flaxseed to a salad; it will not affect the taste.

In cases of gastritis it is recommended to put three tablespoons of flaxseed in a jug of water at night and the next day to drink two 8-ounce glasses throughout the day.

The same remedy can be used as a gargle for sore throats (laryngitis, pharyngitis), but if you add honey, it is even better. Flaxseed is one of the nutrients that appear in the Bible. Flax seeds in water, without heating, help to defecate babies and adults.

*11-pag. 128-131. *12p. 130, 140-141, 165-169.

Garlic

(Allium sativum)

A nutrient found in the Bible, garlic helps treat skin conditions, digestion, and is antiviral, antifungal, and antibacterial. In later sections of this book, you will see how garlic is used to treat many ailments.

Garlic has been used in cooking and for health problems for thousands of years. Following the invention of the microscope, the ability of garlic to kill bacteria was known, when Louis Pasteur placed garlic cloves on a plate containing bacteria and was able to observe through the microscope that garlic had eliminated bacteria.

The nutrients present in garlic include folic acid, iron, magnesium, phosphorus, potassium, selenium, zinc, vitamin B1 (thiamine), vitamin B2 (riboflavin), vitamin B3 (niacin), and vitamin C. All these substances bound together and together with 21 other photochemicals, all working in synergy, produce a result that only Nature can achieve. Garlic has shown positive results in cases of colds, cardiovascular diseases, prevention of blood spills, cancer, allergies, aging, angina, arthritis, bronchitis, diabetes, earache, high blood pressure, high cholesterol, nervous disorders, and infections.

A recent study in England showed that consuming garlic supplements during pregnancy can prevent increased blood pressure and protein retention in the urine. Studies have also shown that such supplements can help achieve a significant increase in body weight in babies destined to be born under normal weight. The study was conducted by Dr. D Sooranna, Dr. J Hirani and Dr. I Das at the Academic Department of Obstertrics & Gynaecology at Chelsea & Westminster Hospital in London, UK. They concluded that although delayed growth and high blood pressure are very complex problems, taking standardized garlic supplements during pregnancy can decrease the chances of pregnancy and birth complications.

Ginger

(Zingiber officinale) Other names: jengibre dulce (Puerto Rico), gan jian (pinyig, si seco), shen jian (pinyin, si fresco), sunthi, nagara (sankrit, si seco), ardraka (sankrit, si fresco).

Ginger is a stimulant, diaphoretic, expectorant, carminative, antiemetic and analgesic. It is recommended in cases of cold, flu, indigestion, vomiting, belching, abdominal pain, laryngitis, arthritis, hemorrhoids, headache and chest pains. In Traditional Chinese Medicine there are several formulas to treat the 'rebellious Qi ' (the spleen does not have enough Qi to help in the process of sending the bolus into the intestines).

I have observed that ginger "alone, without more help" can in many cases eliminate vomiting and reflux. I consider that there is an excessive use of anti-acids that is not only unnecessary but also harmful to health. The stomach needs acid to be able to break down food so that the body can use it, that's how God made us. If the stomach is alkalized for a long time, the body cannot perform its natural function of breaking down food, so many people suffer from so many imbalances named in many ways (there are more than 3000 names of diseases in allopathic medicine), but many are the consequence of lack of acid in the stomach and lack of energy (Qi) of the spleen. I have recommended and with great success cease the antacid and have a ginger tea at lunch and dinner for people who have been suffering from stomach disorders.

*18-p. 10, 15.33-35, 37.78. *13-p. 36-38.

Guava

(Psidium guajaba) Other names: guava, cotorrera guava, Peruvian guava (Cuba), red guava, Chinese guava, Peruvian guava, Peruvian guava, deer guava (Mexico); Guava apple tree (Colombia); worm guava (Nicaragua).

The leaves were used in baths in Cuba as an astringent in the cure of sores and skin diseases and the cooking of logs for diarrhea. The infused leaves are used against indigestion and colds. The guava of Peru is the strongest astringent of all guava varieties.

All varieties of guavas are rich in vitamin C. In the Dominican Republic, ripe guava and pineapple mixed in a shake is used to increase the hemoglobin count in the blood.

Güira Maroon (Guira Cimarrona)

(crescentia cujete) Other names: güira común, güira larga, güira redonda, totuma (Cuba), árbol de las calabazas, cirian, cujete, quiro totumo, tecumate (México), morro, morro guacalero (Guatemala), calabacero, guacal (Costa Rica), calabazo, palo de calabazo, palo de tutumas (Panamá), mate, totumo (Colombia), cutuco, huacal, jícaro de cuchara, jícaro de guacal (El Salvador), higüero (Puerto Rico).

Maracas, drinking utensils and making sweets in which it is necessary to beat are made with the dried fruit.

I will limit myself to a single medicinal use of which I have heard very favorable testimonies of people from Cuba and the Dominican Republic, and it is for respiratory diseases, even the most severe, such as chronic cold and asthma. Make a hole in the güira fruit and add honey to the soft mass of the güira. Wait 2-3 weeks, and take two or three tablespoons per day.

The güira, like many other herbs of the Health Olympiad, does not appear in modern books on herbology.

*9-p. 490-492.

Horse Radish

(armaracia lapathifolia) Other names: mostaza de fraile, rábano de caballo (España).

According to Arias y Costas, "it is diuretic and perhaps antiscorbutic".

It is also used against rheumatism, chronic hoarseness, amenorrhea and leukorrhea.

Parts used: fresh roots.

The radish is very popular in the Dominican Republic where it is not only used naturally but also forms part of commercial syrups that are very popular.

*10-p. 783-784.

Hot water

Putting our feet in a tub, basin, or bucket with hot water is an effective remedy to get warm if we come home after a long walk in the cold or if our feet got cold for any reason like snow shoes, water inlet to the feet, etc. *8-pag. 8-15

In cases of rheumatism, gout or muscle aches, nettle, horsetail, juniper can be added to hot water.

To sedate the nerves: oatmeal, valerian, lemon balm

To regulate the circulation: rosemary, lemon balm or lavender.

In cases of cooling: eucalyptus, thyme, ginger.

Indian Bejuco (Liane savon)

(govania polygama) Other names: Leñatero (región central de Cuba, Fomento, Trinidad, el Escambray), Bejuco de sopla, Bejuco de Indio, Mascapalo, Bejuco de fuego (Puerto Rico), Liane Savon (Estados Unidos), Chewstick (Jamaica y Estados Unidos).

Distribution: Mexico, United States, Dominican Republic (where Mabí is made with it, and it is one of the components of Mama Juana, a very popular tonic offered to tourists), Jamaica (the most abundant is the lupoloid govania), Peru, Brazil and Central America.

This plant has been used as a dentifrice, diuretic, depurative, against the retention of fluids in the body, in cases of stomatitis, influenza, venereal diseases, sores, hypertension. It is used in the preparation of Mabi in the Dominican Republic and to a lesser extent in the eastern region of Cuba.

The author knew this plant by the common name "firewood" (leñatero), which does not exist in botany and then I learned that its most common name is Indian Bejuco and that it is much less abundant in Cuba than in other countries. In my research I knew that it is considered a very good honey plant, without further details, but this plant produces a honey of extraordinary quality comparable to the best that the reader finds delighted, among the dark honeys it does not even have competition. In addition, it is very rich in iron, and blooms during the dry season when the bees are desperate because they find no source of nectar, in August in Cuba.

I urge the reader that if he can contribute to the dissemination of this wonderful plant for his personal benefit, especially if he is a beekeeper, and for the benefit of his country, please do so.

Job's Tears

(Coix lacryma jobi) Other names: Doña Juana, Santa María accounts, tears of Moisés (Cuba), camándulas (Puerto Rico), tears of San Pedro (Colombia), pearl grass (El Salvador), yi ren (pinyin).

The leaves, roots, fruits, seeds are used in Traditional Chinese Medicine. It is considered that the coix has several functions: it stimulates the spleen (the spleen is an extraordinarily important organ in Chinese medicine), it stimulates the lungs, and limits the internal heat (a term in Traditional Chinese Medicine), it eliminates pus, and is a natural diuretic.

I have mixed this herb (seeds) with another herb that in Traditional Chinese Medicine is named fu ling (poria cocos), and turned them into powder and then put them in capsules. I recommended these capsules to people with chronic fluid accumulation and the result was excellent.

The diuretic and anti-rheumatic character of Job's tears is found not only in the seed but also in the leaves, according to Pérez Arbolaes, in his book Medicinal Plants of Colombiap., 64, 65.

*10-p. 549-550.

Laurel

(Laurus nobilis)

In cases of sebum balls or tumors, and cotton balls soaked in a strong bay leaf tea and placed in the affected area, for several hours for several days, and it might dissolve. I had a large ball, about an inch and a half long and three quarters of an inch wide and I don't know how much deep, but it went away after doing what I recommend here. It takes time, it is not a matter of one day to another, but the laurel is used a lot in veterinary medicine to lower the inflammation of the tits of the cows, although in the form of oil, which is an allergen in a high percent in humans. I came up with the idea of trying bay leaf tea, which is not considered allergenic because it is used internally in tea and even for cooking. It was a total success with me.

*9-p. 550-552.

Lemon

(citrus aurantifolia)

Lemon, despite being acidic, has a strong alkalizing effect. I highly recommend a lemon top in a glass of water, alternated with a teaspoon of baking soda in a glass of water to raise the Ph to adequate levels (7.2-7.4 +/-), since I think the acidity is related with a large number of imbalances in which the alkalinization of the body is essential to achieve balance and thereby eliminate diseases and preserve health.

In cases of accidents such as burns with the iron, or in the kitchen, etc., the lemon applied to the affected area avoids blisters and allows the affected area to normalize in a short time. Lemon with honey is very good for cold and diarrhea. Pure lemon juice, or a strong juice with water is effective against fighting pain and soreness in the throat. In cases of diarrhea the lemon is excellent because it is a strong astringent without any harmful side effects. Cough: Lemon can help fight cough. Cuts: Lemon is a natural healing, burns a little, but prevents infections and helps wounds heal quickly. Lemon can help reduce uric acid if we consume it with some abundance for four to six weeks.

In cases of eczema, lemon juice could be helpful. In cases of bad breath the lemon helps for its action in the stomach, where it almost always comes from. Acne: place lemon juice on the affected area, wait 10 minutes and without washing spread honey. Wait 10 minutes and wash with water, repeat the process 3 times per week. Swollen tonsils: drink lemon juice little by little. Stains on the face: drink lemon juice every day, two or three times per day. Liver problems: Lemon is a blood purifier so it helps the liver.

*14-p. 620. *10-p. 563-566.

Lemon Balm

(Melissa officinalis) Other names: melissa, toronjil, cedronela (Spanish)

Lemon Balm is one of the herbs belonging to the mint family such as mint, yerba buena and pennyroyal. The taste in tea, like the other mints, is very pleasant, and has inhibitory effects on some viruses of the herpes family, according to Varro Tyler, Ph.D, who was dean and professor of pharmaceutical studies of natural products at Perdue University in West Lafayette, Indiana, USA.

James A. Duke, Ph.D, one of the most renowned herbal experts in the world recommends lemon balm with other mints on hand (hyssop, oregano, mint, rosemary, thyme, yerba buena and sage) in a tea and placed directly on the skin to use its natural antiviral properties to treat herpes and rash. Like the other mints, lemon balm is effective in cases of digestive disorders.

*10-p. 649-650. *15-p. 18, 53, 162,277-278, 288,257-259, 332, 469,545.

Llantén

(plantago major)

Llantén is a common wild grass in barren and cultivated land found in all Caribbean countries, in Bermuda and throughout Continental America from the United States to South America.

This wonderful plant has many uses either taken in tea or in external use.

"The leaves are slightly astringent and are used in gum ulcers, mild ophthalmic hemorrhages and as a febrifuge" – Gómez de La Maza.

"The leaves are used in eye infections." – Alessandri

"Llantén leaves are used as astringent, in the form of cooking, for gargles. With its distilled water, eye drops are made." – Gómez Palmo

"Fresh leaves are used as poultices for herpes of the face, on the diseased part" – Cainas

The llantén was listed in the Pharmacopoeia of Spain and the United States, and quite possibly in other countries.

In the apitherapy section I referred to the llantén next to the marigold, neem and propolis, all ground (those who want to practice herbology in a professional manner will benefit from a machine for grinding herbs and roots), and mixed with honeybees raw, to treat skin conditions of all kinds. This is my personal contribution, where we include western herbs, Ayurveda, and hive products. This mixture was used in a very serious case of skin condition in which allopathic medicine proved inefficient, and we will show the photos for the reader to judge for himself.

I tried to use the same formula on a friend in my town, Fernando Carrero, who was in a center for the sick and elderly, when there was nothing left to do to treat an infection on his leg, except to possibly cut it off. The administrators informed me that I was not authorized to treat him, and when I asked for authorization they declined. I cannot assure you that the successful result described above would be repeated in Fernando, but my treatment would not have done any harm. A pasty mix of herbs and honey never kill anyone. He died without being given the opportunity to try something new, which is a shame because modern medicine had already given up on him.

*10-p. 570-573. *18-p. 13, 21, 26, 32, 35, 75,179-180.

Lobelia

(lobelia inflata) (lobeliae chinensis) Other names: asthma weed, Indian tobacco, wild tobacco (English), ban bian lian (pinyin):

The lobelia has been used by the Native Americans of North America since before the discovery.

Its most important use is as an expectorant in cases of bronchitis and other respiratory tract conditions. In conditions of any kind that do not respond to treatment, the lobelia, "The intelligent herb," can be included, as the renowned herbologist Michael Tierra often calls it in several of his books.

The definition of "intelligent" is because for reasons we do not always know, it has the desired effect.

Lobelia is an expectorant (helps the phlegm out of the throat and lungs), antispasmodic (eliminates or reduces involuntary muscle movements), and stimulant (substances that increase the body's energy, increase circulation and transmit heat to the body). Lobelia also has diuretic effects, it has been shown in in-vitro studies that it has the property of eliminating or reducing the reproduction of many pathogenic fungi.

*9-p. 568-569. *13-p. 149-150. *12, 16, 28,32-33, 35,153-154.

Ma Chi Xian (Verdolaga)

(Pinyin, as pronounced in Chinese)

It is used to treat urinary tract infections or bleeding. In TCM it is said that it disperses heat, expels toxins, cools blood, stops bleeding (at the end of the book we will explain these concepts but only to those who want to know)

Contraindication: Do not use in cases of pregnancy or deficiency of the stomach or spleen.

It has been used in the prevention and treatment of dysentery. "In clinical studies of thousands of participants it was found that a fresh cooked portulaca (ma chi xian and verdolaga are the same), reduces the incidence of dysentery bacillus in those exposed during an epidemic. It is 90% effective in acute cases and less than 60% in chronic cases." – Dan Bensky / Andrew Gamble

Verdolaga is useful in cases of parasites, whether ingested in cooking or in tablets.

Appendicitis: A study was performed on 31 cases of appendicitis were given cooking a 50% ma chi xian (purslane), and 50% pu gon g ying (dandelion, dandelion English), and only one needed surgery.

JB Gutiérrez says that in Argentina this plant is known as a silk flower. "Its juice, saline and mucilaginous is used as an antiscorbutic and diuretic. Food in raw salads soon corrects belly constipation."

Hieronymus affirms in Diaphoric Plants, "It has been used in tea infusion as a drink in diseases of the bladder, kidneys and liver, in scurvy, vomiting blood, cholera, etc. Outwardly, in poultices it serves against burns and inflammation."

Roxburg says, "its crushed fresh leaves are applied externally in erysipelas and its infusion is used as a diuretic, and internally in hemorrhages."

The coincidence of uses of purslane in Traditional Chinese Medicine, in modern western herbology and in western herbology of the last century is amazing. The author attended a course offered by the well-known Dr. OMD Andrew Ellis in New York City, and my notes on this herb are more or less reflected here, using almost exclusively the experiences of researchers from our continent who know a great deal about how and when to use purslane.

*10-p. 910-911. *13- page 98-99.

Mango

(mangifera indica)

Many authors claim mango's usefulness in naturally treating common ailments.

Juan Tomas Roig recommended it for people with low thyroid because of its high iodine content. Cooking the bark of the mango with schnapps and honey is said to be good for bronchitis and cold.

Gómez de la Maza recommended it for the following: rhinitis, diphtheria, tuberculosis, hemorrhages, bronchitis, dysentery, leukorrhea, and nephritis; in addition, the albumin decreases considerably in certain albuminuria.

According to Drury, the fruit almond is used in India and in Brazil as an anthelmintic.

Standley says the seeds are said to have anthelmintic and astringent properties, the bark also but the bark is also useful for skin diseases.

Grosourdy claims that the leaves are considered for dental remedies, that is, good against toothache, and they tone the gums. With ripe green fruits, the leaves produce a deliciously sweet mixture that is useful in treating weakness or sluggishness of the gastrointestinal organs and other complains that relate to them.

Roig recommends the fruit for constipation and that the resin is useful against cracking when applied to the belly, and against bronchitis, on the chest.

Marabou

(dichrosta chysglomerata) Other names: aroma francesa, espina del diablo (Cuba)

Yes, even the Marabou, the plant that has become a plague with the sad distinction of helping Cuba to no longer be one of the countries with the highest percentage of arable land in the world, as when it was controlled, also the "Aroma" can be used as medicine.

Maza and Roig, in their book Flora of Cuba say that this plant can be used as an antiseptic, and if its decoction is applied to the skin, bacteria is prevented from growing. They also say that it is probably a good astringent, due to the abundance of tannins it possesses. It can be used in cases of hemorrhages and secretions, hemorrhoids and inflammations. Tannin-rich plants are the ones that bees visit the most to make propolis, one of my favorite substances and from which you can find information in the apitherapy section and in the naturopathy section.

*10-p. 624-625.

Marigold

(Calendula officinalis) Other names: mercadela, maravilla, caléndula (Spanish)

Marigold is recommended for exterior use to treat wounds, burns, ulcers and fistulas that do not heal quickly. Inwardly it has been used in gastric and duodenal ulcers, imbalances of the liver and gallbladder, and in heart problems related to heart rhythm disturbances. Marigold is an antiseptic (prevents bacteria from multiplying in the skin), astringent and vulnerable (herbs that help heal wounds and accelerate cell multiplication). If it is about the skin, I always include the marigold, even in Chinese medicine formulas that do not include it because the marigold is a western herb, not part of the Traditional Chinese Medicine.

Mint (Yerba Buena)

(mentha piperita and mint spicata)

Both plants, the yerba buena and the mint belong to the mint family and I think that both can be used for the same uses. Both have a very pleasant taste and similar properties. They are used in cases of colds, fever, sore throats, laryngitis, earache, any type of digestive problem, headache and to calm the mind.

I would like to compete these plants in tea against any medication used against headache. Most headaches are related to the stomach, the real cause of pain. If the cause is eliminated, the symptom disappears, but if the symptom is treated only, the symptom will come back again.

*10-p. 881-883.

Moringa

(moringa oleífera) Other names: Linden flower (it has nothing to do with the linden flower), in the region of Las Villas Cuba, Pearl tree, Bequeta tree, Tree of life, Miraculous plant, Drumstick tree, Horseradish tree, Tree of life (southern United States, Jamaica), Malunggay (Philippines), Muringa (India), Sajina (Bangladesh), La Mu (China).

This fibrous trunk tree, not good for use as wood, can reach up to 10 meters high, although in areas where it is grown it is cut annually to keep them at 1-2 meters to facilitate access to its leaves and branches. Tolerates coastal land, dry, sandy and poor land, but does not reproduce in places where the temperature is too cold.

The nutritional value of moringa is impressive, as well as its therapeutic properties. In Ayurveda medicine and in the Philippines its leaves are used to help normalize blood pressure and blood sugar levels. Studies have shown that it contains:

- 4 times the calcium in milk
- 2 times milk protein
- 3 times the potassium of the banana
- 3 times the almond iron

This plant is rich in vitamin A, B, C, D and E, and in minerals such as potassium, calcium, iron, selenium and magnesium. It also contains abundant amounts of amino acids, something uncommon in plants. In Asia and Africa its leaves are consumed in the form of juice, tea, puree, and other forms of preparation for human consumption. Other parts of the plant such as stems, seeds and roots are also used.

My personal experience is limited to a salad of its leaves, and it is not at all unpleasant to the palate. They told me anecdotes of people from my hometown who benefited greatly from the consumption of the leaf of the Flor de Tilo, as this plant has been known for many years. It is not of recent existence as many mistakenly believe, although it has recently spread its use with its real name, moringa.

The fruits of the moringa reproduce in the form of a pod, such as tamarind. Its flowers are white and I have been told that it is a good honey plant.

Partial list of its nutritional and healing properties:

- Stimulates the hormonal system
- Aid against anemia
- Increase memory and cognitive ability
- Strengthens muscles and bones
- Normalize blood pressure
- Lower blood sugar levels
- Detoxifies
- Protects the liver
- Homeostatic (decreases excess fluids in the body, edema)
- Lower cholesterol
- Increase hemoglobin
- Digestion aid
- Boosts the immune system
- It is an anti-oxidant
- Decreases migraine and headaches

- It helps you lose weight
- It helps eliminate or decrease hemorrhoids

United Nations organizations have been given the task of helping to propagate this plant to fight hunger in areas of extreme poverty since it can be grown even in the worst soils with relative ease.

Oats & Oatmeal

(Avena sativa)

Oatmeal is an excellent food, it tastes very good especially if it is prepared with a pinch of salt and honey and cinnamon are added. Recent studies show that it helps lower blood cholesterol levels. It is also used in cases of weakness, depression, menopause, to tone the stomach and spleen, to increase sexual appetite in men and women, worry, anxiety, palpitation, impotence and insomnia.

Okra

(abelmoschus esculentus) Other names: cancha (Colombia), naju (Panama), quingombó, quiabo (Brazil).

Applications: "Valuable as an emollient and demulcent, also diuretic. It is used in colds. The capsules fresh, crushed, like the leaves form good emollient poultice." – Dr. Gibson.

"The okra is a refreshing and emollient food, excellent food for the convalescent and for those who are good and healthy, is perhaps the richest substance in mucilage of the flora of the Antilles" – Grogurdy.

*10-p. 781-782.

Oregano

(oreganum vulgare)

Oregano oil is a strong antiseptic that has the property of destroying fungi, bacteria, ulcers, skin infections, eliminates allergies, parasites, worms, candida, dysentery and foot fungus (external use). It is used in liniments in cases of bumps, falls and sprains, not only in oil but in a simple tea as well.

*10-p. 690-691. *19-p. 129-130, 253, 260,269.

Papaya

(Carica papaya) Other names: fruta bomba (Spanish), lechosa (Dominican Republic, Puerto Rico, Venezuela), mamón (Argentina, Paraguay).

The cooking of this tender fruit has been used with great success in cases of persistent diarrhea of children and at the time of teething. A burning sensation when urinating may be due to excess protein being passed to the urinary system and this can be solved by simply eating ripe papaya in abundance, for example, replacing a lunch or meal.

Twelve papaya seeds are swallowed as pills throughout the day and act as a strong, very effective vermifuge. On the Island of Guadalupe, the juice squeezed from ripe papayas is prepared after being baked, sweetened and taken in tablespoons to treat a cough, including the most serious cases. M Martínez in his book Medicinal Plant of México says: "It is said that the infusion of flowers is emmenagogue, febrifuge and pectoral, and that the cooking of the leaves is of good effect against asthma."

Eating ripe papaya as the only food at lunch for two or three days can solve serious digestive imbalances. Papaya is rich in vitamins A, C and D and contains very powerful digestive enzymes that help eliminate digestive problems of the most diverse. I have recommended a lot and with great success the abundant consumption of papaya, pineapple, sweet potato and pumpkin against various digestive disorders.

*9-p. 438-439. *14-p. 100-101, 314, 349, 420, 621,658.

Parsley

(petroselinum hortense) (apium petroselinum) (petroselinum sativum)

Cainas, in his book Medicinal Plants of Cuba, claims that in addition to being used as a condiment, the leaves are used for laryngitis. This is done by cooking leaves and branches, boiling them for 10 minutes, and taking the drink several times a day. To strengthen the vocal cords, the thickest roots are chewed raw by extracting all the juice and swallowing it. It is assured that it is very good for singers because it clarifies their voice.

In modern herbology the leaves are used as a diuretic, expectorant, and to eliminate urinary tract infections. All parts of this plant are good for stimulating digestion.

*10-p. 739-740. *14-p. 548. *18-p. 13.35-36, 72,175.

Pineapple

(ananás comosus)

Pineapple is beneficial in cases of indigestion, diarrhea, vomiting, inflammation of the abdomen and edema.

In Costa Rica the consumption of pineapple as a substitute for lunch or food is done with the aim of losing weight.

The enzyme bromelain, present in this fruit, increases digestion and eliminates worms.

Pineapple and grapefruit can leave an unpleasant sensation in the teeth so it is advisable to brush your teeth after eating pineapple or grapefruit.

*10-p. 749-750. *21-p. 33-34, 40, 70-71, 74, 103, 110-111, 114-115, 171, 276, 280-281, 315-316, 373-374, 387, 515.

Plantain (Green Banana)

(paradisiacal muse)

The green banana, chopped on wheels to make chicharritas, ladybugs, chifre (very fine), is fried, then ground and that flour is cooked with milk and is given to children who suffer from diarrhea and heal in several days.

We do not have credible testimonies regarding the effectiveness that is said to have the leaves so we do not include anything about it. Plantain as a food is an excellent nutrient and enjoys great preference throughout Latin America.

*10-p. 768-770.

Pumpkin

(Cucurbita maxima)

Pumpkin seeds are very rich in zinc and are easily absorbed. I believe it is best to add zinc to those who are deficient in this mineral, and that usually occurs in people with a poor appetite. It is also excellent for the health of the kidneys and prostate.

According to Gómez de La Maza, pumpkin seed is a vermifuge to eliminate tapeworm and other parasites.

Other types of squash such as American squash and other varieties already common in the US have similar properties.

Someone who I recommended eating pumpkin seeds consumed it excessively and it affected his digestion. It cannot be consumed as if it were roasted peanuts, it has to be consumed in moderation, about 10 to 15 seeds per day could be enough.

The fruit of the pumpkin is like the sweet potato, very good for the stomach and spleen.

*14-p. 548-550. *9-p. 263-264. *15-p. 445-449.

Purple Basil

(Ocimun sanctum)

In studies conducted at the University of Havana in the 1940s by Dr. Nydia Luthy and Dr. Ortelio Martínez Fortun, it was found that this plant has an antiglycemic factor. In their research they found that the majority of their cases displayed a significant decrease in blood sugar.

The research included children from 10 years to adults over 70 years of age. The publication of the results motivated more than 400 people to go to the Agronomic Station to request purple basil to treat diabetes. Many claimed that the treatment was very effective, and many stopped injecting insulin because it was no longer necessary.

The previous testimony offered by Juan Tomas Roig, who was director of the Agronomic Station of Santiago de Las Vegas, Cuba deserves to be taken seriously, not only for the investigative passion and professionalism of said researcher, but also for the little progress that has been made in combating the disease in the last 60 years.

Rose Apple

(jambosa vulgaris) Other names: manzana rosa (Cuba, El Salvador).

It exists in the Antilles and in Continental Tropical America. It is found in humid places, but especially near rivers and streams.

The root was used against epilepsy, and Tomas Roig was assured that it was very successful. According to Stanley, powdered seeds are used in El Salvador as a remedy for diabetes. Many friends of my youth appreciated the fruit, some do not. This plant, and many others in this book, do not appear in any other work of modern herbal medicine. The reason for being included is due to the fact that these plants that were once used as medicine have been totally forgotten by later generations, and that they treat imbalances that still remain unsatisfactory today through modern allopathic medicine, which is also very expensive. I want to offer many options to as many people as possible considering that if they were successful in some, perhaps many cases, today they can also have satisfactory results in those who venture to imitate, without cultural prejudices, their ancestors.

*10-p. 774-775

Rosemary

(rosmarinus officinalis) Other names: romero (Spanish)

Rosemary was an official drug in the Spanish Pharmacopoeia and was part of popular commercial preparations in the first half of the last century such as Vulnery Species, Balm of Opodeldoc and Agua de Colonia del Codex.

Rosemary contains essential oils of cineole, camphor and borneol, and others.

It is used in the form of tea, to a teaspoon of the herb is added the equivalent content of a cup of boiling water, cover and wait ten minutes before straining it. It is used in cases of indigestion, colds, headache, and in inflammation of the joints and rheumatism.

*10-p. 804-805. *18-p. 27, 37.79-80,187-188.

Sago, Arrow Root

(maranta arundinacea) Other names: yuquilla (Cuba and Puerto Rico)

Sago is a plant native to South America that is good throughout the Caribbean, Central America, Mexico and the United States.

Application: a puree is made from the rhizome of this plant, which is made as cassava starch is made. Sago puree, like malanga, was used as a first solid food given to breastfeeding children and adult convalescent for its easy digestion and assimilation.

It has a pretty pleasant flavor and its cultivation is quite easy. I sowed in the courtyard of my house, when I lived in Cuba, in an inappropriate place next to a wall where I barely received the sun and without any care and still produced.

*10-p. 825-826.

Sarsaparilla

(smilax medica) Other names: zarzaparrilla mexicana , zarzaparrilla from Veracruz.

There are other sarsaparilla species such as those in Honduras,

Costa Rica, Cuba, Ecuador, Spain, Jamaica. In Mexico there are more than 20 species. The legitimate one was supposed to be smilax officialis, but almost all sarsaparillas have the same properties. The one in Jamaica, it is much appreciated, is the smilax spinosa. The one in Spain is the smilax aspera, also very much appreciated.

Cembrano, in his book Medicinal Plants, page 179, and Yonken, in his book Treatise on Pharmacognosy, p. 239, say the root is stimulating, diaphoretic and purifying.

It favors digestion and activates nutrition. It is also recommended to cure eczema and chronic rheumatism.

In modern herbology it is also used as an aphrodisiac, blood purifier, in skin conditions, cancer, digestive problems, rheumatism, hypertension, sexually transmitted diseases, such as gonorrhea, syphilis, etc., to protect the liver and to eliminate bacteria and fungi.

*10-p. 988-990.

Scratchbush

(Urera baccifera) Other names: chichicate (Spanish), chichicastre, jamo (Cuba), ortiga blanca, ortiga de la tierra (Puerto Rico), pringamosa (Venezuela), chichicastle, ortiga de caballo (México), guaina, pringamosa (Colombia)

The following is a testimony of an old friend, Orlando Pinto, who gave me permission me to write his experience with the chichicate. His bout with kidney stones had changed him from being extremely affable and always smiling, to always aching and worrying. Once he took chichicate, he returned to his normal cheerful self. Like all his friends from our hometown in Fomento, Cuba, we witnessed the radical improvement in his demeanor after taking chichicate. His experience occurred at the beginning of the 1960s.

"The pain produced by my kidney stones was unbearable. When I would have the stones removed, I would worry they would return at any moment, and it would always returned in a couple of weeks. I was injected with abafortan and the horrible pain was taken away for a few days, but that was only a temporary relief. People recommended to cook the chichicate, so I went to look for it near the river, in La Poza de la Piedra, because it grows in humid places and they told me that I could find it there. The leaf is like a heart, smooth on one side and with hair on the other. It irritates the skin if you touch it with your hands, so you have to be careful, or wear gloves to handle it. Only the root is used, which emerges from the vine to which it is attached. The cooking of the chichicate removed the stone, made it dust and I urinated it out of my system."

Orlando Pinto currently lives in Hialeah, Florida. *9-p. 374-375.

Sea Grape

(cocoloba uvifera) Other names: uvero (Cuba), sea grape, sea grape (Puerto Rico), beach grape (Mexico, Venezuela), grape (Mexico, Dominican Republic), apple (Mexico), papaturro (Costa Rica), beach uvero (Panama and Costa Rica), uvilla (Dominican Republic), hop-wood, horse wood, pigeon wood, goga de praia (Brazil).

Parts used: the leaves, the fruits, the bark, the root.

The Spanish Pharmacopoeia included the Kino of Jamaica, which was made with parts of this plant and used as an astringent.

According to Gómez de La Maza, "the decoction of the bark and root is astringent, useful in diarrhea and dysentery, and the fruits are astringent."

According to Stanley, "the roots are astringent and the bark has febrifugal properties."

"The bark of the trunk, branches and roots all have astringent, hemostatic, and anti-hemorrhagic properties that are all derived from its astringent condition." – Grosoursy

*10-p. 899-900.

Shepherd's Needle

(biden pilosa) Other names: manzanilla del país, margarita (Puerto Rico), cadillo rocero (Venezuela)

Romerillo is a very common wild grass in any type of land in the West Indies, Continental Tropical America, southern Europe and Asia.

Parts used: leaves, flowers and roots.

"It is used in cases of angina and oral problems, gargling with the tea" – Roig

Pittier H, in Usual Plants of Venezuela says "The cooking of some seeds of this plant is taken in three days for liver disease and soon they are cured."

*10-p. 801-803.

Siguaraya

(trichilia glabra) Other names: ciguaraya (Cuba), lemongrass (Honduras), cañache, teaspoon, chorus, garrapatillo (Mexico), uruca (Costa Rica), sweeps oven (El Salvador).

Parts used: the leaves.

The leaves were used in baths against rheumatism in the first half of the last century, and herbalists and the general population agreed that it was of benefit against that disease. Its internal use was revered by some and contraindicated by others. I think that when in doubt and given nature so many options, it is best to limit the siguaraya to its external use, and not include here the benefits that some gave to its internal use.

*10-p. 855-856.

Soursop (Guanábana)

(Annona Muricata; Graviola; Paw in Portuguese)

There are more than 20 scientific investigations that demonstrated the effectiveness of soursop to kill cancer cells.

For more information, refer to the section Suggestions for Specific Imbalances.

Sweet Potato

(Ipomoea batatas)

Sweet potato is one of the foods with the highest fiber content. It is excellent to improve digestion and to facilitate excretion, strengthens the stomach and kidneys, eliminates skin rashes, and increases body fluids. It also tones the spleen which (according to traditional Chinese medicine) helps send processed foods in the stomach to the intestines.

In cases of very serious chronic stomach imbalances I have recommended a sweet potato and pumpkin diet only and we have obtained very good results.

Tamarind

(tamarindus indica) Other names: tamarind (English)

Dr. Juan Tomas Roig reminds us in his book Medicinal or Poisonous Plants of Cuba the following: "the pulp of the fruit is an official drug of the United States Pharmacopeia." This means that the properties of tamarind as medicine were recognized by the medical community, which are still appreciated today in Asia, Africa and in parts of the Americas.

Modern photochemical studies have shown that tamarind contains tannins, saponins, alkaloids and other nutrients that are active against salmonella and staphylococcus aureus bacteria.

The author has had tamarind bars open outside the refrigerator for prolonged periods of time without being corrupted. If bacteria and fungi do not live in the pulp for so long, it is logical to think that it has anti fungicidal and antibacterial properties. Scientific studies are not always necessary. You and I can also formulate theories and be right.

Pulp tamarind is a moderate laxative with the following properties: anti helminthic (extracts worms), antimicrobial, antiseptic, antiviral, anti asthmatic, astringent, fights skin bacteria, eliminates cholesterol metabolism disorders, is good against colds, fights chronic constipation, treats colic, is good against diabetes, is used in cases of chronic diarrhea, bladder disorders, hemorrhoids, indigestion, leprosy, liver disorders, nausea and vomiting related to pregnancy, itching, rheumatism, inflammation of joints and stones in the urinary system.

According to Stanley, "in Madagascar, the cooking of the bark is used against asthma and amenorrhea, the leaves for intestinal worms and stomach disorders. The pulp, in addition to food has been used to preserve food by its action of repelling micro organisms."

Tamarind is much appreciated in Ayurvedic medicine. Dr. David Frawley and Dr. Vasant Lad, renowned Ayurveda specialists and co - authors of The Yoga of Herbs book include it in their book.

*10-p. 862-864. *21-p. 466,484. *22-p. 216.

Thyme

(thymus vulgaris) Other names: thyme (EU).

My favorite use of thyme is as an expectorant in cases of respiratory conditions and for colds of which produce coughing or sneezing, but it is also used in any type of cold: cough, chills, stomach gases, indigestion and diarrhea.

Verdolaga

(portulaca oleracea) (portulaca parvifolia) Otros nombres: purslane (Guyana), alecrin de Sao Jose, anor crescido(Brasil), flores de seda, flor de un día (Argentina), pusley, purslane, pigweed, hog weed(EU), ma chi xian (pinyin).

Parts used: the seeds and the whole plant.

This is a very common herb in Cuba and in the rest of the Caribbean and in all the temperate and tropical regions of the American Continent and in China, where its use is very extensive in Chinese Medicine.

Watercress

(Nasturtion officinale)

This is another of the nutrients found in the Bible. Renowned herbalist Dr. James Duke, Ph. D includes watercress in his books, The Green Pharmacy and The Herbs of The Bible, also mentioned in his works Gaston Bonnier, Gomez Palmo, R. Grosourdy, JT Roig.

Watercress was part of the Spanish Pharmacopoeia. I have personally recommended it many times and I can say that it is the best of nature for its enormous variety of applications, and because it tastes good in salads. Its applications include: Diuretic, urinary tract cleanser, kidney infections, skin conditions, chills, colds, cancer, asthma, tuberculosis, constipation, bad breath, blood cleanser, excess uric acid, sexual weakness, liver pain, facilitates perspiration, is antiscorbutic according to Selene Yeager is protective of the heart, prevents wrinkles, and decreases the danger of having cataracts.

*11-p. 226-228. *9-p. 223-224.

Watermelon

(citrullos vulgaris)

According to Freise and Roig, fresh seeds contain a bitter principle that is vermifuge. The seeds benefit the kidneys and act as a diuretic. They also dilate the capillaries, thereby lowering blood pressure.

Water melon (the fruit), promotes urine, lubricates the intestines, and benefits the heart, stomach and bladder, according to Henry Lu. The melon, according to Traditional Chinese Medicine, has aphrodisiac effects because it is a Yang tonic that stimulates the kidneys, an organ that is related to sexual activity. The white melon bark is said to treat diabetes and high blood pressure in juice, according to Roig. *10-p. 651-652.

Yagruma

(cecropia peltata) Other names: llagrumo (Puerto Rico), coilotopalo, chancarro, guarimbo, guarumo, guarima, saruma (Mexico), imbauba (Brazil).

In Cuba it was quite popular to use the cooking of yagruma leaves as a breastplate and it was considered very effective. Roig Grosourdy attributes the following properties: astringent, cardiovascular and vasculoarterial, anti-asthmatic, pectoral, compromising and diuretic.

Standley, in Trees and Shrubs of Mexico, says that in Mexico the juice is used as a caustic for the treatment of ulcers and for destroying warts. In South America and Las Antillas it is used for dysentery and venereal diseases, and in a decoction of the new leaves for dropsy, liver disease and asthma. Ashes, according to Barham, were used as a remedy for dropsy. It is also said that the plant has the properties of digital, although its toxicity is relatively low.

Teixeira copy of the Journal of the Scientific Society of Paraguay, the following paragraph of a conference delivered by Dr. Langon, of Montevideo, at the Paraguayan Red Cross, "In 39 cases of pneumonia, treated with fluid extract or with infusion and cooking of cecropia peltata leaves the patients healed perfectly and quickly without resorting to the application of injections of any kind, or the help of other medicines. Important to note is that in most cases, the disease stopped after the third or fourth day from starting treatment. Dr. Mauricio has concluded that as a cardiotonic, yagruma can advantageously replace, in many cases, digital. Given its relative low toxicity, this medicine should be administered with a loose hand. I consider it, said Dr. Mauricio, unsurpassed as a heart tonic in uncompensated heart conditions (in asystole and hypo-asystole, etc.). We must also add its effective diuretic action".

*10-p. 934-936.

4. Methods of Preparing Vegetable Plants

Hot infusion

Leaves, flowers, or stems are placed in a bowl and boiling water or hot water is added, depending on the type of leaf or flowers. Cover the container and wait 10 minutes before pouring the liquid.

Cold infusion

Some plants, such as anamú, have a very strong flavor and it is better to add water to the container containing the plant at the same time and wait a few hours before consuming the infusion.

Cooking or decoction

It usually refers to hard parts of the plant such as roots, stems, barks, which require more time to extract nutrients. One way is to place the plant or plants in a non-aluminum container, add water and put on high heat. When it starts to boil, reduce the heat to very low, cover the bowl and cook for 30-40 minutes and turn off. Wait 10 minutes before removing the lid and strain.

Tea

There are many ways, but we can say that the hot infusion described above can be a valid way. Also in some cases you can place the grass along with the water, put on the high heat and when it starts to boil, according to the delicacy of the part of the plant in question, it goes out with the lid on and you wait 5-10 minutes before straining the liquid.

Tinctures

Put the herbs in a glass bowl and cover them with vodka, whiskey, rum, schnapps or brandy. Keep it in a dry place in the shade, stir the liquid frequently, every other day, for example. After two or three weeks, that's it. If it is a tonic I strain the liquid, I make a tea or normal cooking with the herb, together with the strained cooking with the extract and I add my honeybees. The tinctures lasts for many years, tastes good, and is ready without preparation at the time of consumption. Tinctures made with alcohol are not recommended although they extract more nutrients, some say. The truth is that with this method what is not extracted with the alcoholic beverage is extracted with cooking and the risk of consuming pure alcohol is avoided, many of which are highly toxic.

Compress: Make a normal tea, wet a wipe and apply on the affected area in cases of pain, inflammation, cold-like symptoms, etc. Cover the wipe with a dry towel. The wipe should be quite hot but not too hot, in moderation.

Ointments

They do not carry water, but herbs with oils, beeswax, etc. An ointment easy to prepare and very effective is to put the herbs to fry in lard, and spread when the temperature allows, in the affected area.

Essential oils

They are very difficult to do and require very expensive special equipment. In cases where you want to use the best, I think, is to buy them.

Syrup

Medicinal syrups are made when white sugar is added to a tea or decoction. The simple syrup of the British Pharmacopoeia was prepared as follows: 1 kilogram of refined sugar is added to 500 milliliter of boiling distilled water until the sugar dissolves, then distilled water is added boiling until the total weight is 1.5 kilograms. The absolute severity of the syrup must be 1.33. That was called 66 degrees "Brix Solution"

Then the teas or decoction were dissolved to prepare the medicated syrups.

There are other methods, but basically they all consist of dissolving white sugar in a tea or decoction. The lifespan of the syrup is many years while the taste allows even children to consume it.

5. Plants Properties and Functions

Adaptogen

They help to adapt to the environment, temperature, height, humidity, etc., and to deal with emotional, mental and physical problems.

Examples:

- Maca (lepidium meyenil)

- Chinese ginseng (panax ginseng), ren shen (pinyin)

- Siberian ginseng (eleuthrococcus senticosus), wu jia shen (pinyin)

Note: Siberian ginseng is now called Eleuthero, later adopted by law to the first edition of this book. They argued that this plant does not belong to the ginseng family.

Alteratives

They are purifiers of the blood and lymphatic system, repair body tissues, tend to restore body health by improving nutrition and excretion.

Examples:

- Sarsaparilla (smilax medica)

- Nettle (Urtica dioica)

- Aloe Vera

Analgesics

Eliminate or reduce pain when taken orally, in tea or capsules.

Examples:

- Chamomile (chamomilla matricaria)
- Lobelia (lobelia inflata), ban bian lian (pinyin)
- Willow (salix alba), (salix humboldtiana), (salix chilensis)

Antibacterial

They destroy or decrease the replication of bacteria. They should be taken with some frequency, every one or two hours, for example, so that the elimination of bacteria is greater than their reproduction.

Examples:

- Garlic (Allium sativa)
- Thyme (thymus vulgaris)
- Calendula (Calendula officinalis)

Antibiotics

They destroy or reduce the growth of microorganisms.

Examples:

- Echinacea (Echinacea angustofolia), (Echinacea purpurea)
- Chaparral (larrea tridentate)
- Garlic (Allium sativa)

- Bee Propolis

Antifungal

They kill fungi or reduce their growth.

Examples:

- Calendula (Calendula officinalis)
- Llanten, Plantago (plantago major)
- Neen (Azadiracta indica)
- Propolis
- Honeybees

Antiseptics

They prevent the growth of microbes. They usually refer to external use on the skin.

Examples:

- Thyme (thymus vulgaris)
- Oregano (origanum vulgare)
- Calendula (Calendula officinalis)

Antispasmodic

Reduce or eliminate involuntary muscle spasms.

Examples:

- Tribulus terrestris, bai ji li (pinyin), puncture vine fruit (EU), Excellent.

- Lobelia (lobelia inflata)

- Yerba Buena, mint, pennyroyal

- Thyme (thymus vulgaris)

Antivirals

They destroy or prevent the growth of viruses.

Examples:

- Garlic (Allium sativa)

- Echinacea (angustotofolia and purpurea)

- Bee Propolis

Aphrodisiacs

They stimulate sexual desire and power.

Examples:

- Maca (lepidium meyenil)

- Muira Puama (ptecopetalum olacoides)

- Chinese ginseng (panax ginseng), ren shen (pinyin)

Astringent

Constricting, so they can be used in cases of hemorrhoids, hemorrhages, secretions and inflammations.

Examples:

- Horsetail (equisetum arvense)
- Calendula (Calendula officinalis)
- Cinnamon (cinnamomun cassia)

Bronchodilatory

They relax the muscles of the bronchi and thereby facilitate breathing.

Examples:

- Yerba Buena (mentha spicata)
- Peppermint (mentha piperita)
- Anise (pinpinella anisum)
- Lobelia (lobelia inflata, ban bian lian (pinyin)

Carminatives

Eliminate, reduce and prevent gases.

Examples:

- Aniseed (pimpinella anisum)
- Peppermint (mentha piperita)

- Ginger (zingiber officinale)

Circulatory stimulants

They stimulate blood to circulate normally. They are considered cardio-protective as they facilitate the activity of the heart.

Examples:

- Ginger (zingiber officinale)

- Garlic (Allium sativa)

- Cinnamon (cinnamomun cassia)

Diaphoretic

They stimulate sweating and thus help lower fever.

Examples:

- Thyme (thymus vulgaris)

- Peppermint (mentha piperita)

- Ginger (zingiber officinale)

Diuretics

They promote the activity of the kidneys and the bladder, thereby increasing the flow of urine.

Examples:

- Corn fluff (zea mays), Yu mi xu (pinyin)

- Dandelion (Taraxacum officinalis), Dandelion (EU), pu gong ying (pinyin)
- Parsley (petroselinum sativum)

Emmenagogic

They promote menstruation.

Examples:

- Artemisa, sagebrush (artemisia vulgaris), mugwort (EU), ai ye (pinyin)
- Maca (lepidium meyenil)
- Angelica (angelica archangelica), dang gui (pinyin), yang kuei, the same.

Expectorants

They help soften and expel mucous substances from the throat and lungs.

Examples:

- Lobelia (lobelia inflata), ban bian lian (pinyin)
- Anise (pinpinella anisum)
- Bee Propolis
- Thyme (thymus vulgaris)

Hypoglycemics

Lower blood sugar level.

Examples:

- Garlic (Allium sativa)
- Fenugreek (trigonella foenum graecum)
- Gymnema Sylveste

Hypotensive

They lower blood pressure.

Examples:

- Holy thistle (cnicus benedictus)
- Garlic (Allium sativa)
- Bee pollen

Laxative

They facilitate bowel movement.

Examples:

- Aloe Vera
- Flaxseed (linum usitatissimum), Flax Seed (EU)
- Dandelion (taraxacum officinalis), Dandelion (EU), pu gong ying (pinyin)

Vermicidal

They kill and expel worms.

Examples:

- Bomb fruit seeds (papaya)
- Pumpkin Seeds
- Clove (Syzygium aromaticum)

Vulnerary

They promote healing of wounds and areas of irritated skin by accelerating cell multiplication.

Examples:

- Aloe Vera
- Calendula (Calendula officinalis)
- Llanten, Plantago (plantago major)

6. Suggestions for Specific Imbalances

Herbs and formulas of the Chinese herbalist are included here because many can acquire them in Chinese medicine establishments in New York, San Francisco, Los Angeles, Toronto, Madrid, Lima, Mexico City, etc. In addition, they can be obtained online.

The measures do not have to be rigorously accurate, nature is not either. In formulas that do not include measurements, use common sense to achieve equal parts, or desired approximations such as 60%, 40%, 25%, etc., or simply mix without fear of being wrong since herbology, like cooking, is art, not just science.

In relation to nutritional products, a good guide is to follow the manufacturer's instructions when specific amounts are not indicated and common sense in cases of non-encapsulated nutrients such as seeds, fruits, honey, etc.

Arthritis

If you are going to undergo the therapy of bee stings you should consume all the products of the hive: honey, pollen, propolis, royal jelly and if not, they are also beneficial.

Consume:

- Raw honey, unheated, no super filtered or irradiated
- Pollen
- Propolis
- Royal jelly
- Watercress
- Onions

- Basil
- Laurel
- Cardamom
- Marjoram
- Cumin
- Fennel
- Dill
- Ginger. In teas and added to meats
- Black pepper
- Rosemary
- Mint, good grass, Luisa grass, pennyroyal, all mints
- Angelica
- Beet
- Strawberry
- Peach
- Cherry
- Cabbage
- Broccoli
- Cauliflower
- Celery
- Carrot
- Cat claw
- Chlorella
- Star anise and anise (star anise in Mexico)
- Cayenne

- Licorice (gan cao)
- Fenugreek
- Chaparral
- Dandelion
- Linseed oil
- Vitamin E
- Vitamin C
- Niacin
- Pantothenic acid
- Copper
- Manganese
- Selenium
- Zinc, or pumpkin seed

Avoid or reduce as much as you can:

- Synthetic sweeteners, all
- Margarine
- Eggs
- Crabs
- Eggplant
- Milk and cheese

Vegetable oils, except olive, coconut and flaxseed, although the latter is difficult to obtain, at least in NY metropolitan area. The avocado is also very good. Cook with any of them. The others, I think that some are very bad and others are worse, and are related to innumerable health imbalances, not just arthritis.

Avoid aluminum that is already found in cooking salt.

Even in deodorants, aluminum should be avoided.

Avoid cooking with micro waves.

The American & Oriental Herbs arthritis group including Happy Joints (glucosamide / chondroitin complex), Grape seed extract complex, Coral calcium & magnesium complex, Garlic & cayenne complex, Evening Primrose complex and Spirulina have been suggested to people with this disease.

Bee sting therapy, although painful, uncomfortable, intimidating, shows positive results many times since the first sting.

Cold In Its Beginnings

- Lonicera (ren dong teng) 4g
- Forsythia (lian qiao) 4g
- Mint (Bo he) 1-2g

Peppermint can be substituted with yerba buena or yerba luisa. The 3 are from the mint family, have similar properties and very good taste. All teas and boils in this book are recommended with three cups of water unless otherwise specified.

Another formula:

- Fenugreek 3g
- Licorice 3g
- Thyme (thyme) 3g
- 3g eucalyptus leaves

Another remedy:

- Ginger. 3 pieces in a cup of water

Another one:

- Chaparral. ½ teaspoon in three cups of water.

Common Cold

- Thyme (thyme) 2g
- Ephedra (ma huang) 2g
- Anise 2g
- Ginger 4g

Another option

- Fenugreek 3g
- Elder Flowers 3g
- 3g thyme
- Ginger 3g
- Peppermint 3g
- Licorice 2g

And another one

- Elder flowers 3g
- 3g Lavander
- Linden 3g
- Lobelia 1g

- Ginger 5g

Cough, Lots Of Cough

- 2g ginger
- Fenugreek 6g
- 3g anise

Other:

- Yerba Santa 4g
- Lobelia 1-2g
- Schizandra (wu wei zi) 2g

The following formula was recommended to Marcos Hernández of West New York, NJ after he saw several doctors and specialists without positive results. It worked great in this, a very difficult case.

- Apricot seed, bone fruit, damask, apricot in Mexico, apricot seed, xie ren 10g
- Schizandra (wu wei zi) 10g
- Ban xia (pinellia ternate) 10g
- Jie gen (platicodon glandiflori) 10g

My favorite Trikatu formula, very effective Ayurvedic formula, is already in the book but we will repeat it here:

- 1 part dry ginger
- 1 part black pepper
- Aniseed 2 parts

Raw bee honey to form a kind of paste. Take a teaspoon or less when you cough or a little less as prevention until the cough disappears completely.

Dry Cold

- Comfrey root - Comfrey 3g

- Licorice (gan cao) 2g

- Lonicera (ren dong teng) 3g

- Forsythia (lian qiao) 3g

- Lobelia (ban bien lian) 2g

- Eucalyte, 2g leaves

Heartburn

- Coral calcium & magnesium complex

- Chlorella

- Spirulina

Other recommendations:

- Water with lemon

- Water with honeybees

- ¼ teaspoon of baking soda dissolved in a glass of water

- Take organic apple cider vinegar, two tablespoons a day

High Blood Pressure

From AO Herbs:

- Happy Liver Milk Thistle seed extract

- Royal jelly - Royal Jelly

- Evening Primrose oil extract- Primorosa Oil

- Chlorella

- Omega-3 Fish oil & Garlic complex

Further:

- Increase the consumption of celery in soups, raw, in juices or in capsules. Eat a lot of garlic in soups, foods, capsules, etc.

- If you have been taking allopathic medications for pressure you should take 60-80 mg of co-enzyme Q 10 per day because those medications reduce the COQ10 of the cells.

Hives, Poison Ivy

Internal use

- Fan fen (siler) 3g

- Jin jie (schinonepeta) 3g

- Bai ji li (tribulus terrestri) 3g

- Horsetail (horse tail, equisetum) 2g

- Dandelion (dandelion, pu gong ying) 3g

- Ma huang (ephedra) 2g

External use

- Calendula

- Propolis

- Neem

- Llanten, Plantago

- Honeybees

- It has been used with excellent results

Increase Sexual Potency – Kidney and Yin Deficiency

For kidney and kidney Yin deficiency

- Licii berry (gou qi zi)

- Muira Puama

- Sarsaparilla

- Ginkgo biloba

- Damiana

- Morinda (ba ji tian)

- Eucommia (du zhong)

- Maca

- Schizandra (wu wei zi)

Infertility

- Black Cohosh, Cimifuga, Sheng Ma 12g

- Angelica (dang gui) 6g

- Ginger 3g
- Lobelia 1g
- Royal jelly in teaspoons, gel or capsules
- Vitex (agnus castus) in tea or capsules
- Maca, consume as you prefer
- Eat pork kidneys, bulls, rams, etc.
- Season the kidneys with a lot of garlic and ginger
- Eat raspberry
- Take rooster soup
- The above is for both man and women

Insomnia

- Folic Acid
- Calcium Coral & Magnesia
- Vitamin B Maxi complex
- Royal Jelly
- Omega-3 Fish Oil & Garlic
- A tablespoon of honeybees dissolved in water before going to sleep

Itch

Internal use.

The person could have some involuntary movement, or would be unable to extend the tongue without moving it.

- Fan fen (siler) 3g

- Jin jie (schizonepetae tenuifolia) 4g

- Jin yin hua (japanica lonicera) 3g

- Lin qiao (forsythia) 3g

- Mu zei (horse tail) 3g

- Bai ji li (tribulus terrestri) 2g

- Pu gong ying (dandelion) 3g

Low Blood Pressure

- Cayenne

- Ginger

- Cinnamon

- Chinese Ginseng (ren shen)

Low thyroid (Hypothyroidism)

- Algarrobo, I pod (seed), carob in English

- Gentiana (gentian root), (long dan cao) 7g

- Schizandra (wu wei zi) 4g

- Angelica (bai zhi) 4g

- Black Cohosh (black cohosh, cimifuga, shen ma) 4g

- Kelp 3g

- Chinese Ginseng (ren shen) 4g

Put everything in a glass container containing vodka, white rum, brandy, or burning water for two weeks.

Remove the liquid and cook with the herbs with 3 cups of water. Mix the two liquids and add honey. Take two tablespoons a day.

Other beneficial nutrients for low thyroid are:

- Ashwaganda
- Maca
- Guggul
- Fish oil
- Linseed oil
- Avena sativa, very good breakfast, with honey and cinnamon

Multiple Sclerosis

- Linseed oil
- Cod liver oil
- Coconut oil
- Olive oil
- Honeybees
- Bee pollen
- Royal jelly
- Bee Propolis
- Ashwagandha
- Thriphala
- Selenium
- Vitamin E
- B12 vitamin

- Ginkgo Biloba

- Lecithin

- Cold water fish such as salmon, sardines, mackerel

- Papaya (Fruit bomb)

- Pineapple

- A lot of green and not green salad with olive oil. In cases of digestive problems, steamed, boiled, or in soups

- Nuts, if toasted a little, even better

- Eggs

- Rehmannia 6 (Liu wei di huan wan) also known as six-ingredients pill with rehmannia. It can be obtained in pills

- Qi Gong: The simplest, breathe deeply through the nose, counting, 40 times, several times a day

Avoid as much as possible or completely eliminate:

- Tin foods

- Hydrogenated or partially hydrogenated oils

- Margarine

- Milk

- Cheeses

- Beef

- Corn syrups

- Vegetable oils except those indicated above

- Gluten

- All kinds of artificial sweetener, all

- Do not cook anything with micro waves

- Aspirin

- Ibuprofen
- Indomethacin

Nervousness (Increase sexual potency)

- Skullcap (scutellaria lateriflora) 3g
- Sarsaparilla 5g
- Muira Puama 5g
- Damiana 3g
- 3g passion fruit
- Maca 7g
- Schizandra (wu wei zi) 5g
- Eucomnia (du zhong) 5g

Nervousness (To calm the mind – shen in TCM)

- Ginkgo biloba
- Sarsaparilla
- Passion fruit (passion flowers), its leaves
- Verbena
- Skullcap
- Damiana

This formula can serve as an aphrodisiac as in many cases impotence and frigidity are related to the nerves and not to the organs.

Oil for Itching, Inflammation, Wounds and Rashes.

External use.

- Marigold 1-2g

- Plantago (plantain leaf, plantago major) 1-2g

- Comfrey leaf - Comfrey (symphytum officinale) 1g

- Artemis (mugwort, ai ye) 1g

- Heat everything in coconut oil, lard or sesame oil at low temperature.

Painful Urination

- Licorice 3g

- Gotu Kola 2g

- Plantago (Plantein) 2g

- Coriander , 3g seeds

- Nettles (nettle root) 3g

- Uva ursi 3g

- Another option

- Dandelion (4 parts)

- Fenugreek (fennel) 2 parts

- Rosemary (rosemary) 2 parts

- Licorice 2 parts

- Corn fluff (corn zeal, ze may) 2 parts

Poisoning

- Red clover (Trifolium pratense) 3g
- Coriander 4g, seeds
- Dandelion 3g

This formula is excellent, I made it for myself without regret and it worked great, for others I have done it with the measures recommended here.

Rash and Itchy Skin

External use.

- Cooking in three cups of water.
- Frankincen 4g
- Myrrh 4g
- Dandelion (dandelion, pu gong ying) 4g

Skin Itch

- Myrrh 7g
- Neem 3g
- 2g propolis
- Oregano 3g

I have recommended this formula many times, I always have it in spray bottles and I have thought about marketing it with the name

I write to the bottle, "Bye Bye Itching", or "Goodbye Itching", or "Formula for Itching Dr. Martínez "

It lasts effectively for a long time at room temperature since all its ingredients fight microbes, bacteria, viruses and fungi.

This same formula can be used in gargles for sore throats and anti-tartar although I notice that it is not pleasant to the palate because it contains propolis, excellent for the mouth and gums but with an unpleasant taste.

 been a total success.

Sore Throat

- Lonicera Japónica (ren dong teng) 3g

- Fenugreek (fenugreek) 6g

- Eucalyptus, 1g leaves

- Thyme (thyme) 2g

- Peppermint (bo he) 1g good herb is a good substitute 1g

- Licorice 3g

- Forsythia (lian qiao) 3g

- Rosemary (Rosemary) 3g

- 2g ginger

Another option:
- Fenugreek

- Mullein (verbascum thapsus)

- Slippery Elm Bark (slippery elm, North American elm, ulmus rubra, ulmus fulva)

- Anise

- Yerba Santa
- Elder Flowers (sambucas nigra)

Another option:

- Myrrh (mo yao) 7g
- Neem 3g
- Propolis 2g
- Oregano 2g

Another option:

- Forsythia (lian qiao) 4g
- Japan Lonicera (ren dong teng) 4g
- Schizonepetae tenuifoliae (jing jie) 2g
- Peppermint (bo mo) 2g

Another option:

- Comfrey root (syphytum officinale) - Comfrey 1g
- Anise 1g
- Sage (sage officinale), (sage) 1g
- Mullein 1g
- Licorice (gan cao) 1g

I made this last formula for myself, it only hurt my left side, it worked very well.

Sore Throat with Runny Nose

Mysterious Baking, Mysterious Decoction Shen Mi Tang

- Ephedra (ma huang) 6g

- Pruni (xing ren) 6g

- Magnolia (hou po) 6g

- Orange peel (citrus peel, chen pi) 3g

- Licorice treated with honey (zi gan cao) 3g

- Blupleurum (chai hu) 3g

- Cinnamon (cinnamon, gui zi) 3g

In May 2008, I was handed to Shen Mi Tang to a man from West New York, NJ, of Chinese origin, Tai Lee. TL had previously gone to China Town in NYC without getting rid of his imbalance and this formula normalized him with six cups.

Dr. Martinez's Liniment

- Comfrey - Comfrey 5g root

- Turmeric (turmeric) 4g

- Laurel 3g

Put everything in a glass bowl and cover the herbs with alcohol. Wait a week, filter the liquid and cook with the herbs in two cups of water. Join the two liquids. I always have it on hand in spray knobs (sprinklers). You will be amazed at its effectiveness.

Stomach And Lower Belly Pain

- Cardamom) cardamon, frutu amomi cardamomi, bai dou kou) 3g

- Fenugreek (fenugreek seed, trigonella foenum-graecum, hu lu ba, methi in sankrit) 3g

- 3g anise

This formula can eliminate stomach ache instantly.

I usually do it without measuring. On one occasion I gave it to one of those people who have absolutely no faith in the herbs but as nothing took away the pain, he agreed to have a cup, and when he went in half he had no pain.

I cannot assure that it always works, but I have not yet had any experience that has not

Stones – Gallbladder or Urinary Tract

- 3g corn hair

- Nettle (nettle root) 3g

- Dandelion 3g

- Lobelia 1g

- Licorice 2g

- Ursi grape 3g

- Turmeric – Turmeric (jian huang) 3g

- Butcher 'broom (Enebro) 3g

This formula has worked well on several occasions, including a case with a shift to be operated. I must also clarify that with my cousin Arturo, from Florida, did not work and had to operate. I have already mentioned the unquestionable fact that nothing works every time in all people.

7. About Cancer

Cancer has many definitions.

- Replication or reproduction of cells with different, incorrectly formed characteristics that have the tendency to eliminate adjacent cells of nutrients necessary for their normal subsistence, also converting them into cancer cells.

- A toxic or malignant lump

- Disease caused by altered genes that have a DNA that causes other cells to also become cancer cells

- Disease in which cells lose their intelligence and begin to reproduce abnormally causing obstruction and compression of organs, ducts and nerves and decreasing the amount of nutrients available to normal cells

- It's a virus

- It is a bacterium

- It is a fungus

- It is a mental / emotional imbalance

- It is vitamin B17 deficiency

- It is an abnormality of cells that occurs due to vitamin C deficiency

- It is a disease highly related to modern aptitudes, diet, and customs such as lack of exercise, eating processed foods with few or no digestive foods, eating radiated foods, eating foods full of chemicals that do not exist in the food chain and are toxic, consumption of harmful fats extracted from genetically altered products, consumption of tobacco and cigarettes, insufficient consumption of fruits, vegetables, grains, and seeds, among other reasons.

The definitions given here are not the only ones, but they are enough to establish my theory that the Cartesian theory, considered as the only valid form of science, has managed to unnecessarily diminish the attainment of combined methods of therapies against cancer and other diseases. The search for a single treatment against a disease will never work because it bases its search on the Cartesian premise that there is a single truth, in this case a disease and a single cure for those who suffer from the disease. The practice has repeatedly shown that there is nothing that works for everyone because there are marked differences from one person to another, and if any method is condemned because a scientific study shows that it only works X% of the time, it only achieves to eliminate a method that is effective X% of the time.

Conventional medicine has historically condemned unconventional natural remedies, and its followers have been considered people who deserve no respect because they are not scientists, or their work is non-scientific. The first time that a promoter of what was not considered accepted by conventional medicine, who was not entirely considered non-scientific, was in 1970 when Linus Pauling put his book Vitamin C and the Common Cold into circulation. He later suggested that high doses of Vitamin C may be effective in cases of terminal cancer. Pauling won the Nobel Prize in Chemistry in 1954 for his research in quantum chemistry, made huge contributions in quantum mechanics, introduced the concept of electronegativity, showed that the hemoglobin molecule changes its structure when it gains or loses an oxygen atom, proposed that DNA was a triple spiral, conducted important studies in micronutrients and phytochemicals (chemicals in plants), and was recognized as the father of molecular biology, among many other scientific contributions. It is clear to me that high doses of Vitamin C are not always going to be an effective remedy for everyone, but I doubt that never taking Vitamin C is effective.

Next, we will give many options to fight and prevent cancer. I repeat once again, nothing is 100% effective, but more options are synonymous with more hope.

Surgery

In cases of localized cancerous tumors and in easily accessible areas, the best option is, in my opinion, surgery. In cases of difficult access or when the tumor is very large, it is often possible to operate after obtaining a tumor reduction or by other risk reduction methods that modern medical science knows how to handle. Unfortunately, some colleagues in natural medicine believe conventional medicine never works, and they make the same mistake of believing that all conventional methods are ineffective.

Chemotherapy

Conventional chemotherapy is based on chemical treatments. There are various types of chemotherapies. Dr. Simoncini, an oncologist from Rome, Italy, believes that cancer is caused by a fungus and that the best way to eliminate it is by using sodium bicarbonate. His numerous treatments have achieved amazing results.

Dr. Simoncini's theory has many detractors and followers. Dr. Simoncini and his followers believe that his success rate is far superior to that of conventional chemotherapy, while others assure that it is not. What is true is the undeniable fact that sodium bicarbonate alkalizes the blood, and since cancer patients always have acidic blood, sodium bicarbonate can be very useful — either because it eliminates the fungus as Dr. Simoncini says, or because it allows patients to better withstand the dangerous increase in blood acids, a common side effect of conventional chemotherapy.

Currently the efficacy of conventional chemotherapy is much more effective than before. Now the pH of the fully alkaline patient is maintained before and after conventional chemotherapy sessions and the success rate is much higher, possibly due to the sodium bicarbonate used in conjunction with conventional chemotherapy. The truth is that Dr. Simoncini deserves recognition for his influence on conventional chemotherapy, giving more importance to maintaining high levels of alkalinization, even higher than pH 8 in cancer patients. His work has benefitted patients, family members, and society in general.

Radiation

The side effects of radiation are extremely strong. A patient receiving radiation treatment will have a weakened immune system, and there are so many health problems that may follow, including the possibility of the recurrence of the cancer it was treating. I personally know people who underwent chemotherapy and radiation and benefited greatly from consuming aloe and using it externally. I believe everyone who undergoes radiation or chemotherapy can benefit greatly from aloe vera. My method of preparation is found in this book.

Essiac formula

This formula was developed by a Catholic nun from Canada in 1922, named Rene Caisse. It is said that she received it from a woman who 20 years before had received it from an Indian from the Ojibway tribe. With it, her breast cancer was eliminated. So, this formula could be of indigenous origin from the north of the American continent. The formula was popularized with the name Essiac, equivalent to Caisse reading from back to front, perhaps for legal reasons. This formula can be obtained commercially and is perhaps the most popular natural formula against breast cancer. The formula and measures given below are those that I have used in the past and although the ingredients are the same, the measures could be different from those given by other authors.

- Sheep sorrel (rumex acetosella) 3g

- Burdock root (arctium lappa) 10g

- Slippery elm (ulmus fulva) 5g

- Rhubarb root (rheum palmatum) 3g

I recommend cooking in three cups of water and drinking one cup per day, picking the herb in water, and repeating three more cups.

Hoxsey Formula

The history of this formula is interesting. Harry Hoxsey had a daughter who was diagnosed with terminal cancer and was sent home to spend her last days until the inevitable arrived. He used a special formula on his daughter, and she was saved. Some say the formula was delivered by native Indians; others say he helped to formulate it with his grandfather. Because his daughter was saved, Hoxsey, who was a miner and insurance salesman, opened a clinic in Taylorville, Illinois to offer his treatment to the public. He opened several more clinics, 17 in total.

He was accused of fraud, and many of his patients went to court to defend him and show their gratitude to him. His formula, they said, is the reason they were alive. Even though he was not convicted, and had a lot of support from his patients, he continued to receive many lawsuits. He decided to close all his clinics to avoid further persecution.

In 1963, Mildred Nelson, a trusted nurse from Mr. Hoxsey, went to Tijuana, Mexico, where she opened a clinic and continued the same treatment. Many claim that it has saved hundreds of patients, others say that this is not scientifically proven and therefore cannot be considered as a valid alternative. The truth is that many lives were saved thanks to his formula.

Ironically, Harry Hoxsey treated himself with his prostate cancer formula and it did not work. He died from prostate cancer. This confirms my theory that nothing, absolutely nothing is effective

100% of the time, therefore, we must have options without government restrictions or legal pressures.

This is the list of ingredients of the original Hoxsey formula, although the measurements change from one practitioner to another.

- Barberry Bark 5mg

- Buckthorne bark 10 mg

- Burdock root 5 mg

- Cascara sagrada 3mg

- Red Clover 10mg

- Licorice root 10 mg

- Poke root 5 mg

- Prickly ash bark 3 mg

- Stilligia root 5mg

The truth is that the use of the decimal system is gradually becoming widespread in the United States only recently, before there was only the English system with which the first Hoxsey formulas were made, so I think that neither the formula I use nor any another may claim is the absolute original. There are currently Hoxsey formulas on the market that include chaparral, Oregon grape and seaweed (kelp), replacing some original herbs. I cannot comment as to its effectiveness, but I think the prices are exorbitant.

Guanabana / Soursop

There are more than 20 scientific studies that demonstrated the effectiveness of soursop to kill cancer cells. In 1976 Richard D. McCarthy, MD published a report on the US Cancer Centers: Cancer Center Information and Research site, stating that National

Cancer Institute studies showed that soursop leaves and branches were incredibly efficient in destroying certain types of cancer cells.

Also, in 1976 a study conducted at Purdue University, Indiana found that soursop leaves killed cancer cells within six lines of cancers, and was especially effective against prostate, pancreas, and lung cancers. The article, "Paw Paw and Cancer: Annonaceous Acetogenins from Discovery to Commercial Products" was published in the Journal of Natural Products 71.7 in 2008, written by Dr. Jerry L. Mclaughin of the Department of Medicinal Chemistry and Molecular Pharmacology at Purdue University. The Catholic University of South Korea also conducted a study published in the Journal of Natural Products where it says that a chemical found in soursop selectively kills cancer cells in the colon, and that it is 10,000 times more potent than Adriamycin, one of the most common drugs used in chemotherapy.

A study by Cancer Research UK (England) also conducted studies of graviola extract and claimed it had shown that the nutrient can eliminate certain types of cancer cells of the liver and pancreas that are resistant to drugs used in conventional chemotherapy. Soursop is an antimicrobial agent with characteristics like tamarind, capable of eliminating bacteria, worms, viruses and fungi, therefore it meets the conditions required in Dr. Simoncini's theory that asserts that cancer is a fungus, as well as Dr. Royal Rife's theory that cancer is caused by a virus. In any case, soursop is a valid option available to anyone, much better than waiting for a scientific study that can take years to complete. Finally, soursop has significant amounts of vitamin B17, another anticancer agent, especially in the seed.

Herbs Effective Against Cancer

Below is a list of herbs considered effective against cancer. I want to make it clear that when we say that an herb is good for fighting cancer does not necessarily mean that it has similar effects to chemotherapy, that may or may not be true, some purify the blood, others alkalize it, others increase the immune system, etc.

- **Cundiamor** (Momordica charantia): It has been used against all types of cancer. It also helps to metabolize sugars therefore it also helps in cases of diabetes. It has also been used in cases of skin ulcers.

- **Pau D Arco** (Lapacho): It is said to help in cases of solid cancers, in Hodgkin's and in lymphomas. A conventional medical doctor from Brazil supplied Pau D Arco to his wife, a case of terminal cancer and she recovered. In South America, Pau D Arco is very popular, especially in Brazil and Paraguay.

- **Anamú** (Zorrillo, pipi, mapurite, apasote, ipacina): It has been used for prevention and to fight cancer. This herb should be prepared with water at the time, put it in a jar to take the next day. Its taste is very unpleasant, but it exists throughout the continent and may be the best option for some patients.

- **Green tea** (Green tea): Used in any kind, and as a preventative. The incidence of lung cancer among Asian smokers consuming green tea is much lower than that of western smokers. The skepticism of those who attribute this absolute truth to genetic characteristics seems unfounded. It is to deny the undeniable.

- **Ashwagandha** (Withania somnifera): Used for any type of cancer.

- **Cat's claw** (Uncaria tormentosa, cats claw): It is also used against diabetes, tumors and rheumatic pains.

- **Dandelion** (Taraxacum officinales, dandelion, pu gon yin): Dandelion purifies the liver. It has been used in liver, breast, and pancreas cancer.

- **Red Clover** (Trifolium platense): This herb purifies the blood. It is used in any type, especially of the chest and lungs. Red clover, like gingko biloba puts the finest blood so they should not be consumed by those who are taking medications for these effects.

- **Saw palmetto** (Serena serrulata): It is said to be effective in fighting prostate cancer.

- **Broth of Mary** (Silybum marianum, milk thistle) **and Holy Thistle** (cnicus benedictus): Cleans the liver and is used in any type of cancer.

- **Sea herbs** (Sea weed): They have been used against stomach, thyroid, liver and lung cancer.

- **Apricot** (Bone fruit, damask, apricot, apricot, xing ren, Armenian prunus): The apricot kernel is abundant in vitamin B17, which is said to be a powerful anticancer.

Beekeepers & Cancer

Beekeepers have the greatest longevity, and at the same time the lowest incidence of cancer and arthritis among all professions. From all over the world – areas below sea level such as Israel and Holland – great heights such as Puebla, Mexico and Denver, Colorado – very cold areas such as the Swiss Alps – and desert lands such as in Arizona; no matter where they are from, the outcome is the same: low cancer and arthritic rates.

Some beekeepers are whites, Asians, blacks, mestizos, therefore genetics does not have any foundation. There is no research in this regard, but my theory is that something they all have in common is that they consume more honey from bees and receive more bee stings than the rest of the population.

8. About Diabetes

Diabetes has increased in the last 60 years, and continues to increase, reaching levels never seen in the history of mankind. It is actually a syndrome, according to the dictionary, "set of symptoms of a disease", and I would include "more other health problems that may not yet have occurred but may occur."

Let's see part of the list: high cholesterol; food allergy; abnormal insulin; impotence; high glucose levels; obesity; blindness; gangrene; excess fungi; liver failure; heart failure; insulin insufficiency; excess insulin, even if the body does not recognize it (hyperinsulinemia); inability to properly metabolize fats; carbohydrates; the sugars; high triglycerides; vision problems, excess fluids in the body and many other symptoms expressed in modern medical terms that include hyper if something is considered in excess, hypo if something is considered deficient, itis if there is inflammation, and algya if something hurts. (There are over 3000 symptoms listed, including pain in one foot, in the head, in a finger, etc.).

If now it is more and before it was less, the reason has to be that before something was done that is not customary now; or that now something happens that didn't happen before; or a combination of both. The genetic factor is now present, but not more than 40 years ago, the level must be more or less the same, so genetics is not the main problem in the drastic increase in this imbalance.

Let's look at some differences: At the end of the 19th century and the beginning of the 20th century, the United States was perhaps the healthiest country in the world. He had comparatively better health and medical services than most other countries but that is not all.

The oil that was most consumed was flaxseed oil, until in 1950 Archer Daniel's Midland closed its production of flaxseed oil and stopped supplying small producers of flaxseed seeds. The largest source of vegetable omega-3 ceased to exist. Other sources of fat, such as animal fats were considered inferior and harmful by experts.

Subsequently came the unfounded propaganda against olive oil, just when I arrived in the US in 1980, later against coconut oil, and at the same time we were told of the wonderful margarines, vegetable oils, unsaturated oils, hydrogenated and partially hydrogenated oils.

All saturated fats were declared harmful and a primary cause of high cholesterol.

No one among the experts wondered the reason why the Eskimos, with a diet of 60% animal fat remained healthy, and with an incidence of heart problems lower than the rest of the US from generation to generation. Nor were they asked why many Eskimos "matched up" with the rest of the population upon arrival of oil farms in Alaska, when they began to consume the same diet as the others.

Saturated fats are those in which a carbon atom in a fat molecule is bound to two hydrogen atoms, so they are less vulnerable to oxidation. The consumption of modern unsaturated fats is perhaps the first cause of the increase in diabetes in the US and in the rest of the world. I recommend olive oil, coconut, flaxseed (very difficult to get), avocado and animal fats if you do not have the above and avoid all others.

Artificial Sweeteners

Cyclamate, saccharin, aspartame, sucralose, high fructose corn syrup -- all are harmful, toxic chemicals that do not exist naturally in the food chain. Other artificial sweeteners that are not listed are also harmful. This is a practical book, I do not want to theorize more about these artificial sweeteners, I only urge you to seek information for yourself and you will be amazed that these toxins are allowed, and even recommended by those who most influence the health of diabetics.

Natural Sweeteners

Honey, guarapo (cane juice), stevia (widely used in Japan since banning artificial ones in the late 1960s, is used in industrialized countries), panela (scraping), evaporated cane juice, licorice, agave, maple syrup, fruit juice. All of these are better, or at least preferable to artificial sweeteners.

Chemicals In Food

There are more than 1,400 different chemicals added to foods, too many to list them all here. A good way to identify chemicals in food is to read the labels and if you have words that are almost impossible to pronounce, very long, sound like chemicals, or are obvious food colorings like Yellow #40 or Red #12—these ingredients are added to extend the life of the food for many months, and to make food look fresh and pretty.

You must not eat these foods. Good products are the natural ones, those made following the laws of God, those that rot after a prudent time without lasting months with man-made preservatives. If you understand all the ingredients on a food label, if you can identify them as products made in nature, then it is a good food.

Recommendations

Your health depends on you, on your effort in maintaining your own health.

Athletes strive not only for what they do well but also work hard against becoming weaker. In the same way, a diabetic has to have the will to say NO the guava cake sitting in front of him. You may have been told that diabetes has no cure, but others have overcome that imbalance, and you can too if you stop believing in those who tell you that your imbalance has no solution.

The following is a list of formulas in Chinese Medicine available in specialized stores and on the Internet that can be of great benefit to diabetics. Some ingredients may vary, but that will be explained by the practitioner providing the formula. I do not recommend buying herbs and cooking because that is quite complex, therefore we will only include the name of the formula.

Below are the formulas in Pinyin and in English.

*   **SI Jun Zi Tang** (four gentleman decoction, is also known as "four major herbs combination") This formula is recommended when there is a pale complexion, the voice is very low and soft, the arms and legs feel weak and the stool they come out very loose. In theory, we assume that energy (Qi) will increase.

*   **Liu Wei Di Huang Wan** (Six incredients pill with rehmannia, is also named as rehmannia six). This formula could be useful in cases of discomfort and weakness in the lower back, non-severe headache, vertigo, sound in the ears, decreased ability to listen, sweats at night, warmth in the hands and in the soles of the feet. Perhaps also a dry throat with pain, toothache without apparent oral problems. In theory, we assume that Yin (body fluids) will increase.

*   **Jin Gui Shen Qi Wan** (Kidney qi pill from the golden cabinet, also named rehmannia 8). In cases of lower back pain, weakness in the legs, tension in the lower abdomen, you may have difficulty urinating, your tongue may be abnormally pale and inflamed and slightly smoky.

- **Tian Wang Bu Xin Dan** (Emperor of heaven's special pill to tonify the heart). In cases of anxiety, insomnia, sleep with shock, inability to think well and concentrate, bad temper, you forget things, dry stools, red and bare tongue, without the white cover. Calm the mind (shen), increase the Yin of the heart.

Herbs, nutritional supplements, and foods that could be useful (of course it doesn't have to be all at once, everyone should know that it is available, which could be useful)

- Aloe
- Cundeamor (bitter melon)
- Fenugreek
- Dandelion
- Laurel
- Psylium seeds
- Escarole (chicory)
- Figs
- Gymnema sylvestre- Shardunika
- Blueberry-Blueberries
- Devil 'club
- Licorice
- Oats
- Turmeric- Curcuma
- Siberian Ginseng(now eleuthero)
- Myrrh
- Juniper berries
- Barberry
- Solomon's seal (yu zhu)
- Amalaki-gokshura

- Guggul
- Neem
- Charantia
- Purple basil
- Coconut oil
- Grama
- Ground pomarrosa seeds
- Tamarind
- Zinc (pumpkin seeds is a good alternative)
- Vitamin C
- Chromium
- Niacin
- Magnesium
- Vitamin B complex
- Carnitine
- Gamma linoleic acid
- Real palm root

American & Oriental Herbs Diabetes Group:

- Omega-3 Fish Oil & Garlic Complex
- Coral Calcium & Magnesium Complex
- Garlic & Cayenne Complex
- Chlorella
- Organic Coconut Oil

9. My Nutritional Formulas

All products listed in this section are produced by my company American Oriental Herbs & Natural Nutrients (AOHNN). We use the following products because their ingredients are all natural, and because they are identified in the Bible. They have proven their effectiveness over the years. Our products come in many forms — hone-based products, tinctures, tablets, and herbal teas. We make every product following local and federal guidelines.

Chlorella

"To be absolutely sure of something, we have to know all or nothing about it" - Olin Miller

Chlorella is a green algae that can quadruple every twenty hours, something that no other plant can achieve. Chlorella has a high concentration of chlorophyll, a pigment that is the main source of photosynthesis, a phenomenon that allows living organisms to obtain energy from sunlight. It also contains a varied amount of minerals, vitamins, and amino acids. Chlorella has the mysterious Chlorella Growth Factor, CGF (Chlorella Growth Factor), mainly a derivative of a nucleic acid that has been widely studied in Japan. Chlorella is also a hormonal simulator with characteristics that allow tissue repair, even in cases of tissue ulceration or destruction in which the damage has resisted other methods.

The chlorella is extraordinarily abundant in RNA and DNA, both responsible for directing the renewal, growth, and repair of tissues and in the cleaning of toxins at the cellular level and in the regulation of the acid-alkaline balance of the blood, helping to reach the PH a its optimum point of 7.2 on the scale. Chlorella is considered one of the best substances in the protection and cleaning of the liver as well as the waste disposal system of the body.

Chlorella is a complete food that contains vitamin C, vitamin E and most minerals. It improves the immune system, prevents ulcers, helps in pregnancy (when cell reproduction is needed to the fullest), helps to fight cancer, can reduce high blood pressure and cholesterol, accelerates the activity of T cells and B cells, the best defenders against viruses and bacteria, helps control sugar levels in cases of diabetes, hypoglycemia and body weight gain and helps control depression.

Our chlorella is 100% organic, pyrenoid chlorella, the most abundant in CGF.

Coenzyme COQ10

COQ10 is a natural compound that found in each of the body's cells and is essential in the production of cellular energy. COQ10 is fundamental in the proper functioning of the mitochondria, part of the cell where most of the cellular reactions of respiration and transformation of glucose and lipids (fats) occur.

There is a clear statistical correlation that demonstrates that people with heart problems have a low relative amount of COQ10 in cardiac muscle cells, so it is considered very beneficial to supplement the body with COQ10, especially considering that this coenzyme has no negative effect in normal doses of 40-60 mg per day.

Many people have consumed COQ10 for the following benefits: heart problems, prevention of heart attacks, hypertension, migraine prevention, Parkinson's disease, weight reduction, diabetes, kidney imbalance, and to restore COQ10 levels to those who use drugs such as statins (cholesterol lowering agents), because these drugs reduce the levels of COQ10 in the cells.

Coral Calcium & Magnesium Complex

In the United States, calcium is considered the prime mineral that helps maintain healthy teeth and bones. It is added to countless foods and products of all kinds that have consumers believing they maintain sufficient levels of calcium in their body.

However, the reality is different.

Calcium deficiency in the United States is alarming. There are so many people who suffer from low bone tissue density and use drugs to increase it. Many people break their bones upon an inconsequential fall as if their bones were made of crystal. Why?

Most products that include calcium are a waste because the body does not absorb nor assimilate it due to their ineffective formulas. Calcium does not work alone in the body. It needs other substances such as magnesium and vitamin D.

Our Coral Calcium & Magnesium Complex includes 500 mg of coral calcium along with magnesium, vitamin D, and vitamin C for easy assimilation and absorption.

Our coral calcium is not the typical inorganic stone that the body fails to use but organic coral calcium that is used by the body in more than 400 vital reactions. It really does help maintain strong teeth and bones.

Coral Calcium & Magnesium Complex also helps alkalize the body, at pH levels of urine and saliva above 6.5, which helps avoid common problems in people with high levels of acidity, such as cancer, diabetes, tuberculosis, high blood pressure, lupus, arthritis, chronic diarrhea, fatigue, headache, insomnia, nervousness, among other things.

Evening Primrose Oil

"Success is often the result of taking bad steps in the right direction" - Al Bernstein

Primorose seed oil contains GLA gamma-linolenic acid, a substance recently investigated that can relieve different conditions such as itching, eczema, chronic skin problems, high cholesterol, high blood pressure, problems in the joints and pre-menstrual problems and female problems in general. For this last condition it is considered a highly recommended specific.

Another substance contained in this oil, linoleic acid, an essential fatty acid provided by plants, protects against skin, heart, rheumatoid arthritis, cancer, and multiple sclerosis problems.

Our Evening Prim rose Oil Extract contains 1000mg of the original oil extracted to contain 730mg of Cis-Linoleic Acid (LA) and 90mg of Gamma Linolenic Acid (GLA)

Flaxseed Oil

"And the priest shall put on his linen garment, and shall wear linen underpants on his body; and when the fire has consumed the burnt offering, he will set aside the ashes from the altar, and put them by the altar."- Leviticus 6:10

Flax seed (flaxseed oil) contains a high amount of omega-3, a substance closely linked to the protection of the heart. Omega-3 keeps the skin with the required moisture and can help retain calcium in the cell which benefits the formation and maintenance of strong bones. It also helps lower total cholesterol and triglyceride levels and helps prevent blood clots. Flax Seed (flaxseed) is considered a specific nutrient for the prevention of blood clots, one of the leading causes of death and permanent sequela in the world. Studies suggest that omega-3 may lower homocysteine levels.

A study in Holland showed that glucose intolerance, which indicates a pre-diabetic condition is much less common among those who consume high doses of omega-3.

Flaxseed oil also contains omega-6, omega-9 and other fatty acids that are very beneficial to our body.

American & Oriental Herbs & Natural Nutrients emphasizes the need to maintain adequate homocysteine levels, although this is something almost unknown to the general public, and little considered by the medical community. There are many studies that correlate homocysteine with cardiovascular problems, and we intend to be pioneers in what we know will one day be a well-known risk factor.

Homocysteine is a sulfide-containing amino acid. A level of 5 to 15 micro moles per liter is considered normal. Between 16 and 30 it is considered moderate. From 31 to 100 it is considered intermediate and above 100 micro moles per liter it is considered severe. Heart disease and heart attacks in people with normal cholesterol levels is common and very rare in people with normal homocysteine levels.

We recommend our Organic Flax Seed Oil, Omega-3 Fish Oil with Garlic Complex, Vitamin B Complex and Folic Acid to maintain adequate homocysteine levels, in addition to the many other benefits these nutrients provide.

Folic Acid

"If you want to get enemies, try to change something" - Woodrow Wilson 1856-1924

Folic acid is the most stable of all the B vitamins. It is closely related to the normal production of white blood cells. Folic acid has been used with extraordinary success in pregnancies, this being perhaps its best-known use, and with justified reason: it is vital in cell reproduction, growth and development of the fetus during pregnancy. It has been statistically proven that it achieves a reduction of between 60% and 100% in birth defects. Low levels of folic acid are associated with imbalance such as cancer, poor memory, insomnia, depression, dementia, delirium, irritability, osteoporosis, and anemia.

Garlic and Cayenne Extract – Garlic & Cayenne Extract

"We remember the fish we ate in Egypt for nothing, cucumbers, melons, leeks, onions and garlic; and now our soul dries up; for nothing but this mana sees our eyes "- Numbers 11: 5-6

Garlic has been used in cooking and for health problems for thousands of years. Garlic has shown positive results in cases of colds, cardiovascular diseases, prevention of blood spills, cancer, allergies, aging, angina, arthritis, bronchitis, diabetes, earache, high blood pressure, high cholesterol, nervous disorders, and infections.

Cayenne has been used in cases of diarrhea, cramping, heart protection, circulatory problems, arthritis, indigestion, colds, flu, prevention of stroke and headache.

Our Garlic & Cayenne Extract complex is a 100: 1, 300mg extract of odorless garlic and a 4: 1 extract of 150mg of cayenne.

Grape Seed Extract

"I am the true vine, and my Father is the Labrador. Every branch that does not bear fruit in me, removes it; and everyone who bears fruit cleanses it so that it bears more fruit "- John 15: 1-2

The grape was perhaps the first plant in the Bible to have been cultivated. It appears for the first time in Genesis 9:20. The grape has been an important part of civilization since then.

Recent researchers believe that the consumption of wine in countries whose coasts touch the Mediterranean contributes significantly to the average good health of the inhabitants of those countries.

Our Grape Seed Extract Complex contains 100mg of grape seed and 300mg of bioflavonoids. This powerful combination of antioxidants fights the formation of free radicals, reactive molecules that bind to other molecules causing damage to healthy cells. Free radical formation is the starting point for many diseases, including two of the leading causes of death in the United States and in the world: heart disease and cancer.

Many studies show that a combination of antioxidants provides greater protection against free radical formation than a single antioxidant.

Other studies show that antioxidants can protect against the following imbalances: arthritis, herpes, hypertension, rheumatism, tuberculosis, blood clots, eye problems, impotence, varicose veins, eczema, cellulite, allergy, and aid in the natural formation of collagen.

Remember that an ounce of prevention is greater than a ton of problems.

Happy Joints – Glucosamine & Chondroitin Complex

Glucosamine sulfate is a simple molecule of easy absorption very important for the body since it is a precursor of articular cartilage. Glucosamine also promotes the influx of sulfur into articular cartilage. The body's ability to produce glucosamine decreases with age and this results in the type of natural jelly responsible for preventing bone friction decreases dramatically, which can result in joint discomfort and arthritis.

Chondroitin sulfate is a structural component of cartilage that provides essential characteristics for bones to have strength and the ability to resist pressure. This substance is also essential in the structural consistency of cartilage and bone tissue. Loss of cartilage chondroitin sulfate is considered a major cause of the development of osteoarthritis.

Flavonoids are pigments responsible for the color of many fruits and flowers, these pigments are very effective in reducing inflammations, stabilizing the structure of collagen and preventing the formation of free radicals due to their powerful antioxidant properties.

Manganese deficiency causes weak tissues in tendons and bone tissue. Studies show that women who suffer from osteoporosis have low levels of manganese compared to women who do not suffer from such disease.

Our Happy Joints formula has the right balance and proper nutrient mix to help fight cartilage and bone imbalances.

Happy Liver – Milk Thistle Seed Extract

"Thorns and thistles will produce you, and you will eat field plants" - *Genesis 3:18*

This plant, known in Spanish as Cardo de María or as Milk Thistle (silibum marianum), is perhaps the most revered herb in the world for good liver health.

There is widespread consensus among herbalists, nutritionists, and naturopaths regarding the unquestionable, wonderful properties of this herb to cleanse the liver of toxins. On the other hand, Milk Thistle prevents blood clots, reduces fever, lowers blood pressure, lowers menstrual problems, acts against stones in the urinary system and helps eliminate respiratory problems.

Our Happy Liver is a 4: 1 extract of 1000mg of milk thistle seed without additives. This product can be effective in cleaning the liver of toxins and increasing the level of glutathione in the liver by up to 35%. Clinical studies demonstrate the correlation between the level of glutathione in the liver and the ability of that organ to eliminate toxins.

Happy Prostate – Saw Palmetto-Saw Palmetto Complex Extract

"Each generation laughs at past fads, but religiously follows the new" - *Henry David Thoreau*

Saw Palmetto (seroa repens) is a moderate diuretic and aphrodisiac with recognized efficiency for the urinary system and sexual imbalances such as impotence, frigidity, elongated prostate and ovarian problems.

Pumpkin seed (curcubita pepo) (pumpkin seed) contains a high amount of zinc that is easily assimilated and absorbed, which has been shown in studies that can help reduce the size of the prostate.

Pygeon africanum reduces the size of the prostate in acute inflammation, improves urine flow, and like saw palmetto, reduces the effect of potent forms of testosterone on the prostate, thereby avoiding the risk of getting prostate cancer

Uva-ursi (arctostaphylos uva ursi) is very beneficial in cases of infection in the urinary system as well as in cases of chronic urinary imbalance.

This product consists of four nutrient extracts that have been shown to provide protection to the prostate in a scientifically crafted mixture.

Hive Marvels Bee Pollen Complex

"The really important thing is never to stop asking questions" - Albert Einstein

There is a general tendency in a branch of modern science that tends to connect the effect of isolated substances contained in a nutrient to its therapeutic effect.

Another trend considers that although said isolated substance has such characteristics and benefits, the whole is more important (be it grass, seed, etc.), than the importance given to one or more of its isolated elements.

In the case of beehive products, we have to infer that synergy, that is, all elements together are the reason for the result for the simple reason that all products produced by bees have a lot of variety in color, taste and composition from one sample to another, since bees process what nature puts at their disposal to produce honey, bee pollen, time of year, etc. Yet, despite these changes, the benefits of these products remain . It is interesting to know that beekeepers, large consumers of hive products, generally live a longer and healthier life than the rest of the general population of their countries, including doctors.

Pollen is rich in vitamins B1, B2, B3, B5 (pantothenic acid), B6 and B12.

It also contains vitamins A, C, E, folic acid and carotenoids, as well as amino-acid and protein (20%). It contains Routine and natural hormones HGH (human growth hormone) and minerals such as calcium, copper, iron, magnesium, phosphorus and more. Pollen is not considered an herb or a vitamin but a food that has the most essential nutrients to preserve life, so much so that a person can live by feeding on pollen only for 20-30 years if he did not have another food.

Pollen has been used in cases of allergies, anemia, appetite regulator, asthma, chronic fatigue, low immune system, impotence, infertility, ulcers, prostate problems, menopause, kidney problems, weight control, high blood pressure and for Improve sports results.

Hive Marvels Bee Pollen Complex also contains royal jelly and propolis, both substances with extraordinary health maintenance properties.

Lecithin

"Health, like freedom, is not a passive product that can be sent or bought, but an active process, a continuous search for coherence. It is to navigate our own ship in the sea, without reaching a certain port as the final destination. Health is no more the absence of a disease than freedom, the absence of interference in our lives. Both things involve identifying and overcoming obstacles "- Harriet and Efrem Korngold. Between Haven and Earth, p 383

Lecithin is a phospholipid that is essential in the biological function of the cell membrane.

It has been shown that this phospholipid is beneficial for the circulatory system, the nervous system, cognitive ability (ability to learn and memorize), and to keep the liver healthy.

Our lecithin is from soybeans and contains 61% phosphates which ensures greater protection to the cell membrane.

Omega-3 Fish Oil and Garlic Extract

Fish and garlic have played a very important role in the welfare of mankind for thousands of years. Both provide delicious and nutritious foods that give us strength and health. Yes, cheers!

Global statistics clearly reflect the correlation between high life expectancy and high consumption of fish and garlic. A study in Norway showed greater health in general and greater heart health among people residing near the coast, where fish consumption is very high compared to people residing away from the coast where consumption of said food is much smaller.

The economic income and the wealth of the land does not seem to be a determining factor. Inhabitants of Greenland, with 0% of productive land and very cold climate as well as inhabitants of the Pacific Islands, with high temperatures and reefs and volcanoes on land, enjoy of a long and healthy life. But do not worry! You don't have to move to the middle of nowhere!

Our Omega-3 Fish Oil and Garlic provides nutrients that have clearly demonstrated its benefits in scientific studies, empirical evidence, and personal testimonials. It can lower cholesterol and triglyceride levels, can inhibit the formation of stones, reduce the concentration of calcium and protein in bile, can lower blood pressure, reduce the risk of heart attack, could inhibit the expansion of cancer cells especially in the prostate, colon and breast, can reduce the abnormal heart rhythm, and reduce inflammation.

Organic Coconut Oil

"When you find that you are on the side of the majority, it is time to pause and reflect" - Mark Twin 1835-1910

Coconut oil was a common ingredient used for baking and frying. This happened a long time ago, when diabetes, chronic fatigue, hepatitis, lupus, inflammation of the arteries, and other ailments were not even remotely common as today. At that time, doctors did not see a single case of childhood diabetes.

The absence of coconut oil is not the only reason to blame for the many common health problems man Americans face today. However, the exchange of coconut oil, flaxseed oil, butter, and lard for more modern, low-fat, vegetable oil-based margarines can be the cause of why the United States, the healthiest country in the world at the beginning of the 20th century, is now the world leader in obesity, heart disease, cancer, and many other diseases in this beginning of the 21st century.

Coconut oil is medium-chain saturated fat. "Saturated" fat means that each carbon atom in a fat molecule has two hydrogen atoms attached to the carbon atom and for that reason they are not vulnerable to oxidation and free radical formation that occurs in unsaturated fats. Coconut oil is the main source of cooking oil in the Pacific Islands, the Philippines, India, Indonesia, Thailand and Sri Lanka and its inhabitants have low cholesterol, low incidence of heart disease and a generally normal body weight.

There are many health benefits associated with coconut oil. Some have been scientifically proven, others empirically, and others come from anecdotes — all worthy of consideration and respect. The general health benefit of so many millions of people for hundreds of years is very difficult to deny simply for lack of documented studies. Coconut oil has helped people in cases where many attempts with other medically-prescribed remedies did not achieve their goal.

Coconut oil can be used to aid in heart health, cancer, diabetes, strengthening the immune system, promoting weight loss, increasing the absorption of nutrients and minerals, fighting bacteria and viruses, herpes, bladder infections, gum problems, addressing frail skin and hair, and much more!

Our coconut oil is organic. High doses of up to 12 gels per day are totally harmless.

Propolis – Bee Propolis

Propolis another of the wonderful nutrients produced by bees. It has been used for thousands of years for its therapeutic properties against imbalances such as allergies, herpes, sore throat, nasal congestion, respiratory problems, flu, colds, coughs, wounds, ulcers, skin problems, acne, fatigue, burns, cancer, anemia, dental care (some good pastes contain propolis), liver cleansing and digestive problems.

Hundreds of studies have proven that propolis is a powerful antibiotic and anti-virus that acts against countless types of bacteria, viruses, fungi, is anti-inflammatory and anti-oxidant (eliminates free radicals). The hive is a living example of this wonderful substance. Bees apply propolis to the hive and in doing so manage to protect the hive from invaders such as bacteria, mold, yeasts, fungi, even insects and other predators. Such protection cannot be obtained in clinics or hospitals, no matter how often they apply the most powerful disinfectants.

Propolis is a mixture of wax and resins collected by bees and perhaps metabolized by bees by adding certain enzymes. Propolis contains an undetermined number of compounds that have not been isolated in the laboratory but work in synergy with known substances that are all vitamins with the exception of vitamin K and 13 of the 14 basic minerals that our body requires.

American & Oriental Herbs & Natural Nutrients distributes propolis with calcium and propolis alone, both of excellent quality and purity.

Royal Jelly

Royal jelly is a secretion produced by the hypo-pharynx and the jaw gland of worker bees between 5 and 10 days old. This is the only nutrient given to queen bee cells and the only food the queen bee consumes.

The queen bee weighs 200mg and measures 17mm, compared to 125mg and 12mm of the worker bee. The queen bee lays between 2000 and 2400 eggs a day, with a weight equivalent to 200 times its own weight. This wonderful substance contains a large number of different vitamins, 20 amino acids, DNA, RNA, gelatin, a precursor to collagen, hormones and unknown substances that have never been isolated in laboratories.

Royal jelly has been used as a nutritional supplement for the immune, cardiovascular, endocrine, and nervous system.

Royal jelly can help in more imbalances than any other substance on earth. The list includes: menopause, impotence, infertility, hormonal imbalance, endocrine system disorders, viral infections, bacterial infections, low immunity, skin wrinkles, skin tags, chronic fatigue, heart problems, high cholesterol, high blood pressure, control of weight, retarded growth, eczema, ulcers, mononucleosis, anabolic support (athletic ability), diabetes, depression, arthritis, lack of memory, cancer, liver problems, Parkinson's disease, anemia and spleen infections.

Sounds a lot like a miracle, right? Well, the queen bee can live 5 years while the worker bee lives 6 weeks, and both come from the same type of egg, everything is equal except one thing, food, Royal Jelly.

Spirulina

"Each generation laughs at past fashions, but religiously follows the new"
- Henry David Thoreau

Spirulina is a single-celled algae found in fresh water of lakes and lagoons. Bible scholars speculate that spirulina may have been the food that God provided to the Israelites when they faced the desert for 40 years on their journey from Egypt to the Promised Land. The Aztecs used spirulina as one of their main food sources more than 500 years ago. Today it is available as food in more than 70 countries. Spirulina has a long history in the African country of Chad, where no significant adverse reaction has been noticed even in high amounts of its consumption.

Spirulina is a complete protein that contains all the essential amino acids, vitamins B, C and D and minerals such as calcium, chromium, copper, iron, magnesium, manganese, phosphorus, selenium, sodium, and zinc.

This algae is abundant in chlorophyll and beta carotene, it is rich in GLA (gamma linoleic acid), a fatty acid that is useful in cases of joint problems. It contains an abundance of enzymes essential for digestion and is considered to greatly increase the immune system. Spirulina helps alkalize the PH in the blood and bring the PH closer to its ideal point between 7.2 and 7.4 on the acidity scale. It is also an excellent toxin cleaner that manages to stop the spread of viruses.

Our spirulina is 100% Spirulina Pacifica, certified organic.

Vitamin B Maxi Complex

"The Seven Emotions are joy, anger, worry, sadness, sorrow, fear, impression. The Seven Emotions can cause diseases and similarly, imbalances of the internal organs can cause The Seven Emotions "- Yellow Book of the Emperor. Internal Medicine classes. 300 BC

All living organisms, be they from the vegetable kingdom or the animal kingdom, need vitamins for their growth, for their health, and even for maintaining their life. They use sunlight, carbon dioxide, water, and minerals from the sub-soil to meet their vital needs.

The sub-soil does not contain the vitamins that it used to have 50 to 80 years ago due to modern agricultural practices that prioritize mass production over nutrition. The land no longer rests for 7 years as was customary practice back then. Lack of vitamins in the soil implies lack of vitamins in food which results in a lack of vitamins in the body of those who consume such foods.

All vitamins are necessary. Vitamin B2 is essential for cellular oxygenation, and to avoid itching, cracked lips, burning eyes, and sensitivity to light. B6 helps prevent or reduce confusion, depression, and mouth ulcers. Vitamin B6 is necessary for normal activities of the nervous system, for normal functioning of hormones, and for the formation of red blood cells.

Studies show that heart disease and myocardial infarction are linked to high homocysteine levels than to other risk factors such as cholesterol. Studies have also shown that vitamin B6, in combination with two other B vitamins, vitamin B12 and folic acid, can control elevated homocysteine levels in the blood. We recommend the consumption of Vitamin B Maxi Complex and our Folic Acid to keep this risk factor under control.

10. My Tinctures

Most of our liquid extracts and tinctures are made the old-fashioned way as recommended by the Eclectic School Philosophy. The Eclectic School Philosophy stablished the practice of selecting doctrines from different systems of thought without adopting the whole parent system for each doctrine. In cases of herbs that they never used; we utilize a simple proportion to resemble as similar as possible their technique.

All our liquid extracts are from plants from some of the most recognized companies of the USA, in most cases organic, but not always. We believe that old not necessarily equal inferior. That is the reason that we listen to Mozart, Beethoven, Bach, and Chopin and eat the apple pipe of gramma. We utilize also modern ways to do our herbal extracts. We believe that it is not a good idea to discriminate methods that has been proved to be effective or entire herbal systems such as Ayurveda, Western, Chinese, or Native American. Whatever is good is welcome.

"And God said, Behold, I have given you every herb bearing seed, which is upon all the face of the earth, and every tree, in which is the fruit of the tree, in which is the fruit yielding seed; to you it shall be for food" – Genesis 1: 29

Acacia / Gum Arabic

Acacia Senegal, Acacia Pygnantha, Acacia Decurrents

Ingredients: Acacia Senegal, A. Pygnantha, A. Decurrents, Filtered Water, Premium Grain Alcohol (40%). Dry Herbal Strength 1:4

What is it used for?
Lowers cholesterol levels, keeps blood sugar in check, digestive disorders, alleviate constipation.

Angelica

Angelica Sinensis

Chinese Name: Dang Gui

Other Names: Sankrit: Choraka

Ingredients: Angelica Sinensis , Filtered Water, Premium Grain Alcohol (40%). Dry Herbal Strength 1:4

What is it used for?
Tinnitus, unclear vision, palpitations, moistens the intestines, reduce swelling, helps in menstrual disorders. Channels entered: Heart, Liver, Spleen.

Anis Seed

Pimpinella Anisum

Ingredients: Pimpinella Anisum, Filtered Water, Premium Grain Alcohol (40%). Dry Herbal Strength 1:4

What is it used for?
Stomach complains; dispels gas and flatulence; reduce nausea; cramps.

Ashwagandha

Withania Somnifera

Ingredients: Withania Somnifera, Filtered Water, Premium Grain Alcohol (40%). Dry Herbal Strength 1:4

What is it used for?
Increase strength and vitality, improve sexual debility, nerve exhaustion, loss of memory. los of muscular energy. insomnia, anemia.

Astragalus

Astragalus Membranaceous

Chinese Name: Huang Qi

Ingredients: Astragalus Membranaceous, Filtered Water, Premium Grain Alcohol (40%). Dry Herbal Strength 1:4

What is it used for?
Protect the liver against many different toxins, increase the inmune system to fight chronic fatigue and infections. Channels entered: Lung and Spleen.

Bay Laurel

Laurus Nibilis

Ingredients: Laurus Nibilis, Filtered Water, Premium Grain Alcohol (40%). Dry Herbal Strength 1:4

What is it used for?
Used in cases of high blood sugar. insomnia, migraine, earache, arthritic and rheumatic pain.

Bee Propolis

Bee Propolis

Ingredients: Bee Propolis, Premium Grain Alcohol (40%). Dry Herbal Strength 1:4

What is it used for?
Fight bacteria, fungi and virus; acne; colds; burns; anti-inflammatory; anti-oxidant; allergy; herpes; nasal congestion; respiratory complains; catarrh; acne; cancer; dental imbalances; anemia; liver protector; throat pain

Bee Propolis Throat Spray

Bee Propolis

Ingredients: Bee Propolis, Premium Grain Alcohol (40%). Dry Herbal Strength 1:4

What is it used for?
Fight bacteria, fungi and virus; acne; colds; burns; anti-inflammatory; anti-oxidant; allergy; herpes; nasal congestion; respiratory complains; catarrh; acne; cancer; dental imbalances; anemia; liver protector; throat pain

Bitter Melon / Cundeamor

Momordica Charandia

Other Names: Sanskrit: Karela

Ingredients: Momordica Charandia, Filtered Water, Premium Grain Alcohol (40%). Dry Herbal Strength 1:4

What is it used for?
Weight loss; may low cholesterol; high blood sugar; increases digestion.

Black Cohosh

Cimicifuga Foetida, Cimicifuga Daurica, Cimicifuga Racemosa

Chinese Name: Sheng Ma

Ingredients: Cimicifuga Foetida, C. Daurica, C Racemosa, Filtered Water, Premium Grain Alcohol (40%). Dry Herbal Strength 1:4

What is it used for?
Swollen or painful gums, ulcerated gums, painful and swollen throat, menstrual pains.

Black Pepper

Piper Nigrum

Chinese Name: Hu Jiao

Other Names: Sanskrit: Marich

Ingredients: Piper Nigrum , Filtered Water, Premium Grain Alcohol (40%). Dry Herbal Strength 1:4

What is it used for?
Blood sugar control; digestive stimulant; expectorant; constipation; anti-inflammatory. Channels entered: Stomach and Large Intestine.

Black Walnut

Juglans Nigra

Ingredients: Juglans Nigra, Filtered Water, Premium Grain Alcohol (40%). Dry Herbal Strength 1:4

What is it used for?
Treat intestinal worms, help in cases of candida, tonify the intestine, it is a mild laxative, assist in cases of ringworm and fungi infections.

Blood Root

Sanguinaria Canadensis

Ingredients: Sanguinaria Canadensis, Filtered Water, Premium Grain Alcohol (40%). Dry Herbal Strength 1:4

What is it used for?
Coughs, sore throat, skin complains, gum problems, asthma.

Burdock

Arctium Lapa

Chinese Name: Niu Bang

Ingredients: Arctium Lapa, Filtered Water, Premium Grain Alcohol (40%). Dry Herbal Strength 1:4

What is it used for?
Helps the body reduce excess water, reduce pain caused by arthritis and rheumatism, reduce backache. Channels entered: Lung, Stomach.

Calendula / Marigold

Calendula Officinalis

Ingredients: Calendula Officinalis, Filtered Water, Premium Grain Alcohol (40%). Dry Herbal Strength 1:4

What is it used for?
Antiseptic, antiviral, anti-inflammatory, used in all skin complains, vaginitis from candida infections, help in cases of gum infections.

Cardamom

Elettaria Cardamomum

Chinese Name: Sha Ren

Other Names: Sanskrit: Ela

Ingredients: Elettaria Cardamomum, Filtered Water, Premium Grain Alcohol (40%). Dry Herbal Strength 1:4

What is it used for?
May low blood pressure; digestive stimulant; constipation; stomach complains.

Cat's Claw

Uncaria Tormentosa

Other Names: Spanish: Uña de gato

Ingredients: Uncaria Tormentosa, Filtered Water, Premium Grain Alcohol (40%). Dry Herbal Strength 1:4

What is it used for?
Anti-inflammatory, increase the immune system, improves blood circulation, used in cases of Lupus, diabetes and arthritis, anti-tumor, anti-viral.

Cayenne

Capsicum Fratescens

Chinese Name: La Zi

Ingredients: Capsicum Fratescens, Filtered Water, Premium Grain Alcohol (40%). Dry Herbal Strength 1:4

What is it used for?
May relieve pain and inflammation, digestive aid, stimulate circulation, burn fat-based calories.

Celery Seed

Apium Graveolens

Ingredients: Apium Graveolens, Filtered Water, Premium Grain Alcohol (40%). Dry Herbal Strength 1:4

What is it used for?
Natural diuretic, may lower blood pressure, help the digestive system, relieve symptoms of rheumatism and gout.

Cinnamon

Cinnamomum Cassia, Cinnamomum Zeylanicum

Other Names: Sankrit: Twark

Ingredients: Cinnamomum Cassia, C. Zeylanicum, Filtered Water, Premium Grain Alcohol (40%). Dry Herbal Strength 1:4

What is it used for?
Frequent urination, impotence, colds, sinus congestion, blood sugar high, weak back.

Comfrey Root

Symphytum Officinale

Other Names: Spanish: Consuelda

Ingredients: Symphytum Officinale, Filtered Water, Premium Grain Alcohol (40%). Dry Herbal Strength 1:4

What is it used for?
Bone healing; sores; ulcers; increase cell proliferation; reduce lung imbalances.

Echinacea

Echinacea Purpurea

Ingredients: Echinacea Purpurea, Filtered Water, Premium Grain Alcohol (40%). Dry Herbal Strength 1:4

What is it used for?
Anti-oxidant; arthritis; anti-viral; anti-inflammatory; antibacterial; sinusitis

Elder Flower

Sambucus Nigra

Ingredients: Sambucus Nigra, Filtered Water, Premium Grain Alcohol (40%). Dry Herbal Strength 1:4

What is it used for?
Skin conditions, clear mucus, congestions, chronic sinusitis, reduce flu and cold, reduce anxiety.

Fenugreek

Trigonella Foenumgraecum

Ingredients: Trigonella Foenumgraecum, Filtered Water, Premium Grain Alcohol (40%). Dry Herbal Strength 1:4

What is it used for?
Blood sugar regulator; gout; aphrodisiac; cholesterol; increase women milk.

Frankincense

Boswellia Sacra

Ingredients: Boswellia Sacra, Filtered Water, Premium Grain Alcohol (40%). Dry Herbal Strength 1:4

What is it used for?
May reduce arthritis and rheumatism, used for urogenital ailments, may improve memory.

Garlic

Alium Sativum

Chinese Name: Da Suan

Other Names: Spanish: Ajo, Sanskrit: Rashona

Ingredients: Alium Sativum , Filtered Water, Premium Grain Alcohol (40%). Dry Herbal Strength 1:4

What is it used for?
Cold, heart problems, hypertension, high cholesterol, skin disorders, edema, rheumatism, hemorrhoids, kill bacteria.

Ginger

Zingiber Officinale

Chinese Name: Rou Gui / Gen Jiang

Other Names: Sankrit: Andraka (fresh), Sunthi, Nagara (dry)

Ingredients: Zingiber Officinale, Filtered Water, Premium Grain Alcohol (40%). Dry Herbal Strength 1:4

What is it used for?
Colds, indigestion, vomits, abdominal pain, arthritis, hemorroides.

Ginkgo Biloba

Ginkgo Biloba

Ingredients: Ginkgo Biloba, Filtered Water, Premium Grain Alcohol (40%). Dry Herbal Strength 1:4

What is it used for?
Leg cramps, circulatory problems to arms and legs, improves memory and alertness, help in cases of depression.

Gotu Kola

Centella Asiatica

Ingredients: Centella Asiatica, Filtered Water, Premium Grain Alcohol (40%). Dry Herbal Strength 1:4

What is it used for?
Dilates arteries, repair veins, improves circulation, good for nervous disorders, reduce anxiety, improves memory.

Hawthorn Berries

Crataegus Oxicantha

Chinese Name: Shan Sha

Ingredients: Crataegus Oxicantha, Filtered Water, Premium Grain Alcohol (40%). Dry Herbal Strength 1:4

What is it used for?
Improves blood flow to the limbs, increase oxigene supply to the brain.

Holy Basil

Ocimun Tenuiflorum

Chinese Name: Sheng Lou Le

Other Names: Spanish: Albahaca Morada, Sanskrit: Tulsi

Ingredients: Ocimun Tenuiflorum, Filtered Water, Premium Grain Alcohol (40%). Dry Herbal Strength 1:4

What is it used for?
May reduce blood sugar, boost immunity, purifies the blood.

Horny Goat Weed

Epimedium Glandiflorum

Chinese Name: Yin Yang Huo

Ingredients: Epimedium Glandiflorum, Filtered Water, Premium Grain Alcohol (40%). Dry Herbal Strength 1:4

What is it used for?
Impotence, increase sperm production, help the prostate, reduce frequent urination. Channels entered: Kidney, Liver.

Horsetail

Equiseto Hiemale

Chinese Name: Mu Zei

Other Names: Spanish: Cola de caballo

Ingredients: Equiseto Hiemale, Filtered Water, Premium Grain Alcohol (40%). Dry Herbal Strength 1:4

What is it used for?
Edema, kidney stones, gall bladder stones, stomach ulcers, blurred vision, hemorrhoids. Channels entered: Liver, Lungs.

Immortality Herb / Jiaugulan

Gynostemma Pentaphyllium

Ingredients: Gynostemma Pentaphyllium, Filtered Water, Premium Grain Alcohol (40%). Dry Herbal Strength 1:4

What is it used for?
Adaptogen; longevity; blood pressure regulator; inmune enhancement; lower blood sugar; anti-oxidant.

Joint Pain Formula 1880

Black Cohos, Blood Root, Poke Root

Ingredients: Black Cohos (Cimicifuga Foetida), Blood Root (Sanguinaria Canadensis), Poke Root (Phitolaca Decandra), Filtered Water, Premium Grain Alcohol (40%). Dry Herbal Strength 1:4

What is it used for?
Anti-rheumatic and anti- arthritis formula included in the USA pharmacopeia of 1880 and 1890. This combination was recommended by doctors of the las century until the end of the twenties of last century. We use the same exact proportion of the original formula. Ingredients: Black Cohos (Cimicifuga Foetida), Blood Root (Sanguinaria Canadensis), Poke Root (Phitolaca Decandra)

Knotweed Extract

Polyganum Cuspidatum, Hu Zhang

Ingredients: Polyganum Cuspidatum, Hu Zhang, Filtered Water, Premium Grain Alcohol (40%). Dry Herbal Strength 1:4

What is it used for?
Very important in cases of Lime according to Stephen Harrod Burner. Discharges toxins for burns, carbuncles and other skin infection.

Kutsu-Pueraria / Ge Gen

Pueraria Lobata

Chinese Name: Ge Gen

Ingredients: Pueraria Lobata, Filtered Water, Premium Grain Alcohol (40%). Dry Herbal Strength 1:4

What is it used for?
High blood pressure, headache, tinnitus, diarrhea, alleviates thirst. Channels entered: Spleen, Stomach.

Lavender Flowers

Lavandula Offiicinalis, Lavandula Angustofolia

Ingredients: Lavandula Offiicinalis, Lavandula Angustofolia, Filtered Water, Premium Grain Alcohol (40%). Dry Herbal Strength 1:4

What is it used for?
Anxiety; insomnia; digestive discomfort; gases; headaches; muscle spams; convulsions; depression; anti-inflammatory.

WARNING: Do not use if you are nursing, have gallstones, or obstruction of the billary tract.

Lemon Balm

Melissa Officinale

Other Names: Spanish: Toronjil

Ingredients: Melissa Officinale, Filtered Water, Premium Grain Alcohol (40%). Dry Herbal Strength 1:4

What is it used for?
Irritability, anxiety, restlessness, anti-viral, combats herpes simplex, itching and pain.

Licorice Root

Glycyrrhizae Uralencis, Glycyrrhizae Glabra

Chinese Name: Gan Cao

Ingredients: Glycyrrhizae Uralencis, G. Glabra, Filtered Water, Premium Grain Alcohol (40%). Dry Herbal Strength 1:4

What is it used for?
Stop coughing, relieves abdomen or legs pain. Channels entered: All 12 channels, principally the Hart, Lungs, Spleen and Stomach.

Lobelia

Lobelia Chinensis, Lobelia Inflata

Chinese Name: Ban Bian Lian

Ingredients: Lobelia Chinensis, Lobelia Inflata, Filtered Water, Premium Grain Alcohol (40%). Dry Herbal Strength 1:4

What is it used for?
Promotes urination, reduce edema, asthma, bronchitis, coughs. TCM channels affected: Heart, Lungs, Small Intestines.

Lycii Goji

Lycium Barbarum

Chinese Name: Gou Qi Zi

Ingredients: Lycium Barbarum, Filtered Water, Premium Grain Alcohol (40%). Dry Herbal Strength 1:4

What is it used for?
Sore back and legs, impotence, abdominal pain, blurred vision. Channels entered: Liver, Lungs, Kidney.

Maca

Lepidium Meyenil, Lepidium Meyenii

Ingredients: Lepidium Meyenil, L. Meyenii, Filtered Water, Premium Grain Alcohol (40%). Dry Herbal Strength 1:4

What is it used for?
Boots energy, stamina and endurance; adaptogen; increase libido in men and female.

Mint / Peppermint

Mentha Piperita

Chinese Name: Ba He

Other Names: Sanskrit: Phudina

Ingredients: Mentha Piperit , Filtered Water, Premium Grain Alcohol (40%). Dry Herbal Strength 1:4

What is it used for?
Eliminate gas and flatulence, may stop headache, help in cases of stomach and bowel imbalance, relieves diarrhea and constipation, fight cold and flu.

Moringa

Moringa Oleifera

Ingredients: Moringa Oleifera, Filtered Water, Premium Grain Alcohol (40%). Dry Herbal Strength 1:4

What is it used for?
Stimulate the hormone system, help in cases of anemia, increase cognitive function, improve memory, keep blood pressure in check, protect the liver, lower cholesterol, lower blood sugar level.

Myrrh

Commiphora Myrrah, Commiphora Erythrae

Chinese Name: Mo Yao

Other Names: Sankrit: Bola

Ingredients: Commiphora Myrrah, C. Erythrae, Filtered Water, Premium Grain Alcohol (40%). Dry Herbal Strength 1:4

What is it used for?
Alleviates pain from trauma, stimulate the thyroid, help in casas of skin infections. Channels entered: Heart, Liver, Spleen.

Nettle Root

Urtica Dioica

Ingredients: Urtica Dioica, Filtered Water, Premium Grain Alcohol (40%). Dry Herbal Strength 1:4

What is it used for?
Allergy, arthritis, rheumatism, stimulate hair growth, chronic skin imbalance, asthma, anemia, reduce enlarged prostate.

Oregano Leaf

Origanum Vulgare

Ingredients: Origanum Vulgare, Filtered Water, Premium Grain Alcohol (40%). Dry Herbal Strength 1:4

What is it used for?
Cold; flu; kill bacteria, fungus and virus; anti-oxidant; anti-inflammatory; may help to reduce pain; phlegm; congestions

Parsley

Petroselinum Crispus, Petroselinum Sativum

Chinese Name: Dan Shen

Other Names: Spanish: Perejil

Ingredients: Petroselinum Crispus, Petroselinum Sativum, Filtered Water, Premium Grain Alcohol (40%). Dry Herbal Strength 1:4

What is it used for?
Urinary complains, gall stones, kidney stones, sciatica.

Pau D'Arco / Lapacho

Tabecula Impetiginosa

Ingredients: Tabecula Impetiginosa, Filtered Water, Premium Grain Alcohol (40%). Dry Herbal Strength 1:4

What is it used for?
Fungal infections; lower blood sugar; promotes digestion; may help combat cancer.

Pine Pollen

Pinus Radiata

Ingredients: Pinus Radiata, Filtered Water, Premium Grain Alcohol (40%). Dry Herbal Strength 1:4

What is it used for?
Used in cases of Lime; heart imbalances; reduce cholesterol; increase testosterone; eczema; low libido; longevity; support hormonal balance.

Poke Root

Phytolaca Decandra

Ingredients: Phytolaca Decandra, Filtered Water, Premium Grain Alcohol (40%). Dry Herbal Strength 1:4

What is it used for?
Arthritis, rheumatism, swollen and inflamed glands, chronic bacterial and fungal infection.

Pulsatilla

Pulsatilla Chinensis

Chinese Name: Bai Tou Weng

Ingredients: Pulsatilla Chinensis, Filtered Water, Premium Grain Alcohol (40%). Dry Herbal Strength 1:4

What is it used for?
Ease abdominal pain; benefic the digestive and lymphatic systems; anti-ameba; anti-parasitic; antibiotic. Channels entered: Stomach and Large Intestine. Do not use if pregnant or nursing.

Pygeum Bark

Pygeum Africanum

Ingredients: Pygeum Africanum, Filtered Water, Premium Grain Alcohol (40%). Dry Herbal Strength 1:4

What is it used for?
Reduce size of prostate; improve urinary flow; anti-inflammatory.

Rosemary

Rosmarinos Officinalis

Other Names: Spanish: Romero

Ingredients: Rosmarinos Officinalis, Filtered Water, Premium Grain Alcohol (40%). Dry Herbal Strength 1:4

What is it used for?
May help preserve memory, protect against free radical molecules in the body.

Safflower

Carthamus Tinctorius

Chinese Name: Hong Hua

Ingredients: Carthamus Tinctorius, Filtered Water, Premium Grain Alcohol (40%). Dry Herbal Strength 1:4

What is it used for?
Unblock menstruation, alleviate pain. Use for musculoskeletal trauma. Channels entered: Heart, Liver.

Saint John's Wort

Hypericum Perforatum

Ingredients: Hypericum Perforatum, Filtered Water, Premium Grain Alcohol (40%). Dry Herbal Strength 1:4

What is it used for?
Used for depression, calm the mind, reduce uterine cramping, help fight viral infections.

Salvia Root / Dan Shen

Salvia Miltiorrhizae

Chinese Name: Shen Jian

Ingredients: Salvia Miltiorrhizae, Filtered Water, Premium Grain Alcohol (40%). Dry Herbal Strength 1:4

What is it used for?
Irritability, palpitations, insomnia, itching, rheumatism, promote menstrual regularity.

Sarsaparilla

Smilax Officilalis

Ingredients: Smilax Officilalis, Filtered Water, Premium Grain Alcohol (40%). Dry Herbal Strength 1:4

What is it used for?
Aphrodisiac; cleanses the liver; anti-inflammatory; help the skin; increases muscle mass.

Saw Palmetto

Serenoa Repens

Ingredients: Serenoa Repens, Filtered Water, Premium Grain Alcohol (40%). Dry Herbal Strength 1:4

What is it used for?
Reduce prostatic complains; increase libido; reduce stress.

Schisandra

Schisandra Chinensis

Chinese Name: Wu Wei Zi

Ingredients: Schisandra Chinensis, Filtered Water, Premium Grain Alcohol (40%). Dry Herbal Strength 1:4

What is it used for?
Improve circulation, improves vitality, increase sexual vitality, stop diarrhea, reduce frequent urination, help with irritability, palpitation, insomnia and skin disorders. Channels entered: Heart, Kidney, Lungs.

Skullcap / Scutelaria

Scutellaria Baicalensis

Chinese Name: Huang Qin

Ingredients: Scutellaria Baicalensis, Filtered Water, Premium Grain Alcohol (40%). Dry Herbal Strength 1:4

What is it used for?
Headache, red eyes, clear heat and calm the fetus.

Stevia

Stevia Rebaudiana

Ingredients: Stevia Rebaudiana, Filtered Water, Premium Grain Alcohol (40%). Dry Herbal Strength 1:4

What is it used for?
Allergies; blood pressure regulator.

Stinging Nettle

Urtica Dioica

Other Names: Spanish: Ortiga

Ingredients: Urtica Dioica, Filtered Water, Premium Grain Alcohol (40%). Dry Herbal Strength 1:4

What is it used for?
May lower blood pressure; may help with blood sugar control; may help to reduce the size of the prostate; may reduce inflammation. it is a diuretic but it is also high in potassium. Reduce pain and other symptoms associated with prostate enlargement. Stimulate immunity, useful in cases of anemia, neuralgia, arthritis and chronic skin conditions.

The Supreme Tonic To Nourish Earth

Ginseng and Astragalus Combination, Bu Zhong Yi Qi Tang

Ingredients: Astragalus, Astragali Menbranacei, Radix Ginseng, White Atractylode, Licorice, Glycyrrhiza Uralensis, Cimifugae, Black Cohosh, Bupleurum, Bupleurum Falcatum, Filtered Water, Premium Grain Alcohol (40%). Dry Herbal Strength 1:4

What is it used for?
Chronic fatigue; weakness; poor appetite; general tiredness; shortness of breath; disinclination to speak; diarrhea; uterine bleeding and other hemorrhagic disorders; vaginal discharge; impotence; pernicious anemia; thirst for warm beverages; aversion to cold. The above imbalances may occur do to deficiency of the Spleen and Stomach (Earth Element in TCM). Of course, not all of them have to be present. Ingredients: Astragalus (Huang Qi). Astragali menbranacei; Radix Ginseng (Ren Shen); White Atractylode (Bai Zhu); Licorice (Gan Cao) Glycyrrhiza uralensis; Cimifugae (sheng Ma), Black Cohosh; Bupleurum (Chai Hu) Bupleurum falcatum.

Tribulus

Tribulus Terrestris

Chinese Name: Bai Ji Li

Other Names: Sanskrit: Gokshura

Ingredients: Tribulus Terrestris, Filtered Water, Premium Grain Alcohol (40%). Dry Herbal Strength 1:4

What is it used for?
Dispels wind and stop itching; for any kind of skin lesion with significant itching such as hives. also used in vitiligo. May improve libido in men and women, may lower blood sugar levels; may prevent increase in blood cholesterol.

Turmeric

Curcuma Longa

Chinese Name: Jiang Huang

Other Names: Sanskrit: Haridra

Ingredients: Curcuma Longa, Filtered Water, Premium Grain Alcohol (40%). Dry Herbal Strength 1:4

What is it used for?
Pain related to traumatic injury; menstrual pain; anxiety; reduce gallbladder disorders and jaundice.Channels entered: Heart, Lung and Liver.

Valerian

Valeriana Officinalis

Ingredients: Valeriana Officinalis, Filtered Water, Premium Grain Alcohol (40%). Dry Herbal Strength 1:4

What is it used for?
Promotes relaxing sleep, help with insomnia, may lower blood pressure, calm nervous tensions and anxiety.

Verbena

Verbena Officinalis

Chinese Name: Ma Bian Cao

Ingredients: Verbena Officinalis, Filtered Water, Premium Grain Alcohol (40%). Dry Herbal Strength 1:4

What is it used for?
Relieves tension headache, nervousness, sadness, and irritability.
Reduces blood pressure. Channels entered: Liver, Spleen.

Vitex Chaste Tree

Vitex Agnus-Cagtus

Ingredients: Vitex Agnus-Cagtus, Filtered Water, Premium Grain
Alcohol (40%). Dry Herbal Strength 1:4

What is it used for?
Regulates menstrual cycle of women, reduce menstrual pain,
helps with menopause.

Yerba Santa

Eriodictyum Californicum

Ingredients: Eriodictyum Californicum, Filtered Water, Premium
Grain Alcohol (40%). Dry Herbal Strength 1:4

What is it used for?
Expels mucus; dilates the bronchi; used for sore throat; chronic
bronchitis; flu.

11. My Protocols

Acidity (low Ph): Coral Calcium & Magnesium Complex; Chlorella; Spirulina

Acne: Bee Propolis

Allergies: Garlic & Cayenne Extract Complex; Omega-3-Fish Oil & Garlic Complex; Grape Seed Extract Complex; Bee Propolis; Hive Marvels Bee Pollen Complex.

Anemia: Royal Jelly; Folic Acid; Bee Pollen Complex; Bee Propolis; Spirulina

Angina: Omega-3-Fish Oil & Garlic Complex; Garlic & Cayenne Extract.

Anxiety and Stress: Royal Jelly; Vitamin B Maxi Complex.

Arthritis: Happy Joints Glucosamine & Chondroitin Complex; Grape Seed Extract Complex; Coral Calcium & Magnesium Complex; Garlic & Cayenne Extract Complex; Evening Primrose Oil Extract; Spirulina

Asthma: Bee Pollen; Hive Marvels

Bladder Infection: Omega-3-Fish Oil & Garlic Complex; Organic Coconut Oil; Royal Jelly

Blood Sugar Imbalances: Chlorella.

Cancer: Omega-3-Fish Oil & Garlic Complex; Happy Prostate Saw Palmetto Complex; Coral Calcium & Magnesium Complex; Garlic & Cayenne Extract Complex; Grape Seed Extract Complex; Bee Propolis; Royal Jelly; Spirulina

Cardiovascular Condition: COQ10; Grape Seed Extract Complex; Omega-3-Fish Oil & Garlic Complex; Garlic & Cayenne Extract Complex; Organic Coconut Oil; Royal Jelly; Chlorella; Spirulina

Chronic Fatigue: Omega-3-Fish Oil & Garlic Complex; Coral Calcium & Magnesium Complex; Bee Pollen Complex; Bee Propolis; Organic Coconut Oil

Depression: Vitamin B Maxi Complex; Folic Acid; Royal Jelly; Chlorella

Diabetes: Omega-3-Fish Oil & Garlic Complex; Coral Calcium & Magnesium Complex; Garlic & Cayenne Extract Complex; Chlorella; Organic Coconut Oil

Eczema: Grape Seed Extract Complex; Evening Primrose Oil Extract; Royal Jelly; Spirulina; Chlorella

Hepatitis: Organic Coconut Oil; Omega-3-Fish Oil & Garlic Complex.

Herpes: Bee Propolis; Grape Seed Extract Complex; Organic Coconut Oil; Omega-3-Fish Oil & Garlic Complex.

High Blood Pressure: Happy Liver Milk Thistle Seed Extract; Royal Jelly; Garlic & Cayenne Extract Complex; Coral Calcium & Magnesium Complex; Evening Primrose Oil Extract; Royal Jelly; Chlorella; Omega-3- Fish Oil & Garlic Complex.

High Cholesterol: Organic Flax Seed Oil; COQ10; Garlic & Cayenne Extract Complex; Omega-3-Fish Oil & Garlic Complex; Royal Jelly; Organic Coconut Oil; Chlorella

Impotence: Royal Jelly; Bee Pollen Complex; Happy Prostate Saw Palmetto Complex; Grape Seed Extract Complex; Evening Primrose Oil Extract.

Indigestion: Garlic & Cayenne Extract Complex.

Infertility: Royal Jelly; Bee Pollen Complex

Insomnia: Folic Acid; Coral Calcium & Magnesium Complex; Vitamin B Maxi Complex.

Join Disorders: Happy Joints Glucosamide / Chondroitin Complex Evening Primrose Oil Extract.

Kidney Disorders: High Marvels Bee Pollen Complex; COQ10.

Liver Disorders: Happy Liver Milk Thistle Seed Extract; Lecithin; Chlorella; Bee Propolis; Royal Jelly

Low Immune System: Royal Jelly; Bee Pollen Complex; Folic Acid; Organic Coconut Oil; Chlorella; Omega-3- Fish Oil and Garlic Complex; Spirulina; Vitamin B Maxi Complex; Bee Propolis

Menopause: Royal Jelly.

Migraine: COQ10.

Osteoporosis: Happy Joints Glucosamine & Chondroitin Complex; Vitamin B Maxi Complex; Folic Acid

Pancreas Disorders: Folic Acid; Vitamin B Maxi Complex.

Parkinson's Disease: Royal Jelly; COQ10.

Pregnancy Support: Folic Acid; Chlorella; Garlic & Cayenne Extract Complex; Omega-3-Fish Oil and Garlic Complex; Bee Pollen Complex; Vitamin B Maxi Complex.

Prostate Complains: Happy Prostate Saw Palmetto Complex; Omega-3- Fish Oil and Garlic Complex.

Skin Disorders: Royal Jelly; Organic Coconut Oil; Evening Primrose Oil Extract; Organic Flax Seed Oil; Bee Propolis; Omega-3-Fish Oil and Garlic Complex.

Ulcers: Royal Jelly; Hive Marvels Bee Pollen Complex; Bee Propolis; Raw honey; Chlorella; Vitamin B Maxi Complex. Honeybees .

Urinary Disorders: Coral Calcium & Magnesium Complex; Happy Liver Milk Thistle Seed Extract.

Weight Control: Royal Jelly; Hive Marvels Bee Pollen Complex, Organic Coconut Oil.

12. Patient Testimonials

Elia Vega, from Hazleton, Pennsylvania

I saw Elia for the first time in October 2013. Her voice was almost unintelligible, but between her and her relatives I knew that her imbalances included one of the following.

- Lateral sclerosis (Lou Gehrig's disease)
- Cancer near the lungs
- A tumor in the right hip
- A tumor in the spine
- A tumor in the left lung

Life expectancy according to medical science: none. Apitherapy was the last option. I was very worried about her right foot, which was black, a clear sign that blood did not reach that part of the body. Although that did not bother her doctors very much, for me it was of the upmost importance that they do not amputate her foot. On this first visit, 3 bees were placed, one in the right hand and two in the right foot.

Her eldest daughter just started giving her the ESSIAC formula, which I was going to recommend that same day. I also recommended that she drink Red Clover tea (Trifolium pratense) every day.

On the second visit I placed a bee on the left foot, three on the right foot that was already much better in color and one on the right knee which hurt. Elia was in pain everywhere, but the number of bites should be increased gradually.

In subsequent visits we increased the number of bites at points where she had pain, which were many, and points by the area of the tumors. During this time of treatment, she had suffered from digestive disorders, colds, coughs, and other imbalances all of which have been satisfactorily resolved with herbaceous recommendations and with hive products included in the book. As the areas with pain were decreasing the bites were increasing to points around the tumors and when the analysis indicated absence of cancer the bites have been placed in points that help the recovery of movements according to the acupuncture texts of Chinese medicine.

What is expressed here is only a summary of a long process, but the improvement was remarkable, even extraordinary. Elia speaks and everything is understood, stands up and walks with the help of a wheel cane, has gone to the Dominican Republic to visit her relatives twice in the last two years of treatment. Above all, she lived.

It is important to make it clear that Elia is a person of great faith, of great personal courage, full of love for her family and that she enjoys the unconditional support of those around her, none of whom suggest that my treatment was "not scientific."

Finally, I would like to add that Elia recommended a man from her city to communicate with me because he was suffering from Lou Gehrig's disease, like her, but less severe. I never saw him. What happened to him was what doctors predicted was going to happen. Could another happy story have been repeated? Only God can know, but as the saying goes, the worst try is the one that is not done.

María Alexandra, Queen Colombian, NY

I saw María Alexandra for the first time in July 2008. She was suffering from arthritis in a very serious way. She had pain in practically all the joints of her body. She told me that on the subway she would have tremendous pain when holding onto the handrail and would not sit just to avoid having to stand and feel even more pain. Many nights she could not sleep because she was in so much pain and would spend hours pacing from the living room to the bedroom because of it. María Alexandra's suffering is the worst case of arthritis I have seen so far.

On the first visit I recommended avoiding or reducing as much as possible foods that include aluminum (such as some types of salt and many others), margarine, eggs, cheese, milk, hydrogenated or partially hydrogenated oils , crab and eggplant. Not all of the above is harmful but for her it was by the time I told her. I recommended cooking with olive or coconut oil. I told her to consume the hive products like raw honey, pollen, propolis and royal jelly.

Also a long list of beneficial foods for her condition included watercress, onion, mustard greens, turmeric, basil, bay leaf, cardamom, marjoram, cumin, fennel , dill, ginger, black pepper, Horseradish, Rosemary, Mint, Melissa (Lemon Balm), Angelica, Prickly Ash Bark, Beet, Strawberries, Peach, Cherry, Chestnut, Pine nut, cabbage, turnip root, broccoli, cauliflower, anises, cayenne, licorice, Brussels sprouts, celery, carrot, cat's claw, spirulina, Fennel , chaparral, clove and dandelion.

Supplement recommendations: flaxseed oil, vitamin C 400-800 IU, niacin, pantothenic acid 500mg, copper 1mg, manganese 15 mg per day, selenium 200mcg and zinc 45 mg.

The above list was obtained from my many books. Of course, everything cannot be consumed at the same time, but it was useful in that it indicated what could be beneficial for her. During the 15 months of treatment, I provided herbs for different conditions that were presented.

She usually came from Queen on Saturdays, but sometimes she came in the middle of the week because arthritis pain did not allow her to wait. The number of bee stings fluctuated in general from 8 to 20, but there were many more in certain occasions. She said, on this finger, on the elbow, on the right foot, in this hand, in the forearm, etc.

From July 2008 to March 2009 the total number of bites was 616. From the end of March 2009 to August 2009, 215 more for a total of 831. In September 2009 María Alexandra began to place the bees for her account, as I indicated and was placed in September-October 2009, 52 bites. Then she continued, decreasing the number of bites until she left the bites completely.

I have kept contact with her by phone for the last few years and she is living without the pain that tormented her for so long. María Alexandra now follows an allopathic treatment of two medications that are giving her the healthy life she has always wanted.

Apitherapy, holistic medicine, diet and now allopathic medicine was successful in addressing her issues because she had tremendous fortitude to continue her treatment. She did not listen to friends who criticized holistic medicine and had nothing to offer. She saw the success of the treatment herself, and would often reply to critics with, "This is the only treatment that relieves my pain".

Although there is no cure for arthritis, all of the above, plus María Alexandra personal love for her family and desire to live a better life, helped her successfully live a better life with arthritis.

Augusto (Hobey) Álvarez, of Paterson, NJ.

Hobey informed me that he felt pain in two places, his left shoulder and lower back. He had suffered for a long time and was treated by different doctors and specialists, including chiropractors. He took many different pills without positive result. He is a painter, and he said he was able to work with the pain most times, but sometimes the pain was too great that he could not work.

I immediately proposed bee stings to the shoulder and lower back. I told him, as I do all my patients, that there is no guarantee in this treatment or any other treatment. The treatment may work or not, and if it didn't, we would try something else.

He agreed to the treatment and we began right away. I put a bee on his lower back and another on the affected shoulder and bingo! He felt relieve after only a few minutes after we were don't with the bee stings. The results were better than I expected.

Hobey introduced me with his brother-in-law, José Bolívar Fernández, also of Dominican origin and from Paterson, NJ, who suffered from pain in the hands and knees, but was not diagnosed with arthritis. I treated him with bee stings and the pain was taken away for several months. He returned to see me several years later because he felt strong pains again, although with less intensity than the first time. I applied bee stings on his elbows, hands and knees and the pain went away.

Xiomara López García, of Amancio Rodríguez, Las Tunas, Cuba.

Xiomara suffered from chronic painful mouth sores. I sent her propolis capsules and she placed them directly on the mouth sores, sometimes mixed with a little honey. The sores faded. This is not the only case in which I personally have witnessed mouth sores that were removed with this wonderful substance.

JR from Queens, NY

JR is a two-years-and-nine-month-old girl from Queens, NY. JR is the fictitious name I use in this book since I don't have approval from her family to use her real name. None the less, her treatment is worth including in this book.

JR had airway problems with green phlegm through her nose and in her bronchial tubes. The worst was the desperate pain in her ears. Doctors informed her parents that she had to have ear surgery.

I performed the ear cone candling procedure explained in this book. I also gave them a protocol with yerba buena, lobelia, holy grass, lavender, and elder flower. I also suggested to take honey with lemon and water. Some time later I learned that the pain in her ear and all the phlegm went away, and that they did not have to operate.

I must admit that I didn't know the ear cone candling procedure was going to have such dramatic and immediate results. Again, not all treatments work for everyone, and there are no guarantees. If it did not work, then I would have tried something else. I firmly believe that we must trust in and use our own personal experience and our own intuition when dealing with our own health.

I am happy with JR's results, and for the rest of my life I will be incredibly thankful with what God has helped me do as his simple mediator. This is one of the cases that has given me the most satisfaction.

Don Pedro del Rio, from West New York, NJ

Don Pedro had very little circulation in his left leg. He was given injections that had very little results, and in fact had produced the greatest pains he had ever experienced in his entire life. He decided to stop the injections and treat his symptoms with herbs.

I made a mixture of the following ingredients: plantago major, neem, marigold, propolis, and honey to form a thick paste to be placed on the affected area on his left leg all day long. I recommended that he soak his feet in a basin filled with ginger tea. I also suggested to reduce the consumption of meat and milk, and to eat only well-cooked or steamed foods—nothing fried or raw. In less than 3 weeks the leg showed a normal color and his circulation improved.

The Lady of Guatemala, from Union City, NJ

The lady from Guatemala (she asked that I not use her name) suffered from advanced breast cancer, stomach gases, headaches, sweats in the hands, feet and chest, dental problems with swollen gums, irregular menstruation and pain in the left arm.

Doctors told her that she would live no more than 3 months. I assured her that God is the one who decides how long we are going to live. Words have a healing power, especially in those who willingly accept the positive, and a harmful power in those who blindly believe in the negative.

The protocol was extensive. It included a change in her diet, two formulas against blood stasis (which virtually all cancer patients suffer from), remedies to alkalize the body (it is well known that most cancer patients have acidity in the blood), and anti-cancer formulas from those found in this book. Three months passed since she started her treatment. Then a year. Then another. And then 3 more years, far surpassing what her doctors had predicted.

After a few more months of following the treatment, I lost contact with her until years later. In August of 2014, I called her and she came to see me. She was under exclusively allopathic medical treatment. She received some recommendations on that one visit, but she was weak and not very strong in spirit. I never saw her again. I inquired about her, and they informed me that the lady of Guatemala passed away on January 10, 2015.

JS from Union City NJ

JS was 42 years old when he came to me in 2010, and had a lot of issues. He was diagnosed was sever gastric ulcers and a hiatal hernia. He had stomach inflammation after every meal, a frequent burning sensation in the esophagus, and frequent chest pains. Since he was 19 he's had constant headaches and a low libido.

I recommended that he change his diet drastically and gave him a protocol that included pollen, honey, royal jelly, ginger, and a famous Traditional Chinese Medicine formula named Xiao Yao San (Ramblin Powder).

The results were effective, and everything was normalized. JS was very grateful and flattered me by calling me a magician.

Alberto Martínez (myself)

A sore throat is very common, and whenever I get a sever soar throat I give myself the same treatment. It goes away quickly as if by magic with the following decoction.

- Myrrh (mo yao) 7g

- Neem 3g

- 2g propolis

- Oregano 2g

13. Glossary

Acne: It is a skin condition caused by chronic inflammation of the sebaceous glands. It usually appears on the face and back during puberty. Over time it usually decreases or even disappears.

Acupuncture: It is the art, or science of obtaining therapeutic benefits from a sick person or in physical or mental imbalance by inserting needles at specific points on the surface of his body.

Alkaloids: These are nitrogen organic compounds that have alkaline properties and are extracted from vegetables that contain them. Examples of alkaloids are caffeine, cocaine, heroin, morphine, nicotine and quinine.

Allopathic Medicine: The traditional one that mainly focuses on eliminating or reducing symptoms through the use of chemical drugs.

Amenorrhea: Absence or cessation of the menstrual period. There are two types: primary amenorrhea, when menstruation never occurs, since puberty did not occur and secondary amenorrhea, in this case the menstruation began and then stopped occurring.

Antiseptic: Substances that eliminate microbes when they come into contact with living tissue or on the skin, reducing the possibility of infection or putrefaction.

Antiseptics should be distinguished from antibiotics that eliminate microorganisms in the body, and from disinfectants that eliminate existing microorganisms in non-living objects such as tables, windows, mirrors, etc. Some antiseptics can destroy microbes while others prevent their cell multiplication by creating an adverse environment to them.

Antispasmodic: Substances that eliminate or reduce involuntary muscle movements.

Aphrodisiac: It is a substance that increases potency and sexual desire.

Apitherapy: Apitherapy is the art and science of using hive products for therapeutic purposes, including honey, pollen, royal jelly, bees, wax and bee venom.

Arthritis: Inflammation and joint pain.

Asystole: Complete absence of electrical activity in the myocardium.

Bronchitis: It is an inflammation of the bronchi, located between the lungs. This inflammation can be caused by a bacterial infection or other causes.

Demulcent: A viscous substance that exerts a local protective action, as do the mucous membranes in the mucous membranes.

Diaphoretic: Substance that induces sweat.

Diuretic: A substance that promotes the activity of the bladder with which they manage to increase the flow of urine.

Duodenum: It is the part of the small intestine that connects it to the stomach through the jejunum.

Emmenagogue: Establishes the menstrual flow of women.

Emollient: It is a substance for external use that has the property of softening or relaxing an inflamed part of the body, especially the skin.

Empirical: Knowledge based on experience and observation of facts.

Expectorant: Helps get phlegm out of the throat and lungs.

Fistulas: Abnormal connection between two organs that are not normally connected.

Fungi: They are not plants or animals, although they share certain characteristics with both. Fungi are parasites, which feed on living things and come to produce diseases in them. In the case assigned to us, the human body , the fungi mainly attack the skin and specifically the toes and nails.

Gastritis: It is an inflammation of the stomach lining.

Goiter: It is the enlargement of the thyroid gland. The most common cause is due to insufficient iodine in the diet.

Gout: It is a disease that is believed to be caused by the accumulation of crystals of urate salts (uric acid) in different parts of the body but especially in the joints, soft tissues, and kidneys. Gout attack produces severe pain that usually begins with the big toe.

Hemostatic: Means used to stop bleeding.

Herbology: Also known as phytotherapy, is the study and use of plants and their extracts for medicinal purposes.

Herpes: It is a condition that affects the skin and sexual organs produced by a virus. It is usually transmitted by sexual contact.

Hippocrates: Father of modern, natural medicine original of present-day Greece.

Holistic Medicine: Belonging to holism, a trend or trend that analyzes the events considering multiple interactions that characterizes them, and not just one as is usually the case in allopathic medicine which is highly influenced by the Cartesian Theory. The paradigm of allopathic medicine is totally different and, in our days, unfortunately almost irreconcilable with the traditional one.

Homocysteine: It is a sulfurized amino acid that is related to heart attacks and strokes.

Hyposistolias: Abnormal condition of the cardiac organ due to its dilation, weakness of the heart, rapid pulse, abnormal noise or other causes.

Laryngitis: inflammation of the larynx that affects the normal tone of the voice.

Moxa or Moxibustion: therapy that uses the application of heat at acupuncture points.

Naturopathy: It consists of different types of practices or therapies using elements obtained from nature that are intended to maintain or restore health.

Parasites: or worms: they are organisms that multiply within the intestine and produce a wide range of health problems.

Pharmacopoeia: Compilation of formulas of substances with real or assumed sanitary properties. They were edited from the Renaissance until the beginning of the 20th century including medicinal herbs, and then they have eliminated all natural alternatives to give way only to chemical drugs. There are countries that support the inclusion of natural substances in their pharmacopoeia but these are very isolated cases and are always subject to criticism and accusations in international organizations.

Pharyngitis: Inflammation of the throat or pharynx that causes a sore throat and its cause is due to an infection caused by bacteria or viruses.

Pinyin: It is the Mandarin's transcribed phonetic system, that is, the way a word is pronounced in Chinese using the Latin alphabet.

Psoriasis: Chronic condition of the skin that is characterized by dryness, itching, redness, slight elevation of skin points covered by white sores among other features.

Qi Gong: Modality of breathing exercises and slow movements carried out in order to "cultivate and balance the Qi", in other words, cultivate and balance the body's energy.

Qi: It is pronounced "chi", it is life energy. You can say that life exists when there is also energy. Breathing, talking, sleeping, thinking, seeing, etc., is achieved only when there is energy (qi) in the body. Prenatal Qi is acquired from parents, it is related to inheritance characteristics, what is now known as DNA and the acquired Qi which is obtained from air, water and food.

Rebellious Qi: or rebel Qi, is called when the Qi of the spleen does not have enough strength to send the bolus down and vomiting, bad taste in the mouth, belching, acidity, etc. happens

Saponins have a wide range of biological activity, such as antiviral, anti-cancer, anti-inflammatory, and diuretic. In the industry they are used in the manufacture of soaps.

Saponins: These are compounds that have a complex structure formed by a hydrophilic steroidal core and a hydrophilic part consisting of monosaccharide units.

Spleen: The spleen is an organ that is located on the left side of the body, above the stomach and below the ribs. It is about the size of a fist and is part of the lymphatic system. In Western medicine it is said that you can live without it since other organs will do some of their functions, although it is recognized that without the spleen the body decreases part of its ability to fight infections since this organ contains the white blood cells that fight against the germs and destroys dead, aged and damaged cells. In Traditional Chinese Medicine the importance given to the spleen is much more extensive than what it receives in Western medicine.

Stigmas of corn: The stigmas of corn or corn are the hairs, hairs or beards of these (fluff in Cuba). They can be yellow, golden, brown or almost black. They are a natural diuretic that helps clean the urinary tract. It is prepared in the form of tea, infusion, or cooking.

Stomach ulcers: It is a lesion or hole in the membrane that covers the stomach or duodenum (first part of the small intestine), caused by a bacterium named Helicobacter Pylori (H pylori).

Tai chi: Martial art of Chinese origin used as a form of self-defense and as a means of maintaining good health and increasing longevity.

Traditional Chinese Medicine: It is based on an experience of millennia where the observation of the phenomena is analyzed in depth, in a very wide way but without giving too much importance to why but to what to do to achieve the balance of the imbalance or existing imbalances through methods that in practice they are effective such as the use of herbs, acupuncture, moxa, tui na, etc.

Tuina or Tui Na: Modality of massage therapy of Chinese origin that uses the theory of the flow of Qi through the meridians for specific therapeutic purposes, is not a generalized relaxation treatment such as Swedish massage.

Vermifuge: Substance that expels intestinal worms.

Yang tonic: Substance or substances that increase the potency of the kidneys, spleen and heart.

Yin tonic: Substance or substances that restore body fluids.

14. Bibliography

1-BEE PRODUCTS: Properties, Aplications, and Apitherapy
Edited by Avshalom Mizrahi and Yaacov Lensky, 1997

2- HONEY: The Gourmet Medicine
By Joe Traynor 2002

**3- HEALING FROM THE HIVE: Bee Pollen, Royal Jelly,
Propolis and Honey**
By Rita Elkins, M.H 1996

4- APITERAPIA PARA TODOS
Tercera Edicion Ampliada y Revisada, 2007
Por Moises Asis

5- HEALTH AND THE HONEYBEE
By Charles Mraz 1995

6- THE BIBLE OF BEE VENON THERAPY
By Bodog F.Beck, M.D 1997 Edition

**7- BEE WELL BEE WISE: With Bee Pollen, Bee Propolis Royal
Jelly**
By Bernard Jensen, Ph.D. 1994

**8- La Terapéutica Naturista Aplicada a las Afecciones,
Trastornos y Enfermedades más Frecuentes**
Por Mannfried Pahlow, Licenciado en Farmacia, Cuarta Edición
1992

**9- PLANTAS MEDICINALES, AROMATICAS O VENENOSAS
DE CUBA (Part 1)**
Dr. Juan Tomas Roig. Segunda Edición 1993

**10- PLANTAS MEDICINALES, AROMATICAS O
VENENOSAS DE CUBA (Part 2)**
Dr. Juan Tomas Roig. Segunda Edición 1993

11- HERBS OF THE BIBLE: 2000 Years of Plant Medicine
By James A. Duke, Ph.D. 1999

12- HERBAL REMEDIES
By Asa Hershoff, N.D and Andrea Rotelli, N.D 2001

13- MATERIA MEDICA CHINESE HERBAL MEDICINE
By Dan Bensky and Andrew Gamble. Revised Edition 1993

14- HEALING WITH WHOLE FOODS: Asian Tradition and Modern Nutrition
By Paul Pitchord, Third Edition 2002

15- THE GREEN PHARMACY
By James A.Duke, Ph.D 1997

16- THE COCONUT OIL MIRACLE
By Bruce Fife, CN; N.D 2004

17- COCONUT OIL FOR HEALTH AND BEAUTY
By Cynthia Holzapfel and Laura Holzapfel 2003

18- THE WAY OF HERBS
By Michael Tierra L.Ac; O.M.D 1998

19- HERB BIBLE
Earl Mindell, R.Ph; Ph.D 2000

20- CHINESE TRADITIONAL HERBAL MEDICINE: MATERIA MEDICA AND HERBAL RESOURCE
Dr. Michael Tierra L.Ac; OMD, AHG and Lesley Tierra, L.Ac, AHG 1998

21- LA FARMACIA NATURAL
James A.Duke, Ph.D 1998

22- THE YOGA OF HERBS
An Ayurvedic Guide to Herbal Medicine 2001

23- ENCYCLOPEDIA OF NATURAL MEDICINE
Michael Murray, ND and Joseph Pizorno, ND, Revised Second
Edition 1997

**24- CHINESE NATURAL CURES: Traditional Methods for
Remedies and Preventions**
By Henry C. Lu 1999

**25- TREATING CANCER WITH HERBS. An Integrative
Approach**
Dr Michael Tierra. L.Ac; N.D; AHG 2003

**26- THE PRACTICE OF CHINESE MEDICINE: The Treatment
of Diseases with Acupuncture and Chinese Herbs**
By Giovanni Maciocia 1994

27- INSULIN: OUR SILENT KILLER
By Thomas Smith, Second Edition 1998

28- FORMULAS AND STRATEGIEST
By Dan Benski and Andrew Gamble 1990

29- CHINESE HERBAL SECRETS: The Key to Total Health
By Stefan Chmelik 1999

30- JOURNAL of the AMERICAN APITHERAPY SOCIETY
Excellent magazine with recent information on apitherapy
research worldwide

31- BEE CULTURE
Magazine dedicated to beekeeping but occasionally includes
articles related to apitherapy and herbology.

32 – TRADITIONAL MEDICINE IN GHANA
By Kofi Bobi Barimah and Okyere Bonna 2018

15. List of Distributors

The following list of distributors allows you to purchase patented herbs and formulas without the need for certification or license of herbalism, although some of them do require it.

Mountain Rose Herbs
www.mountain rose herbs.com
PO Box 50220
Eugene, OR 97405
1 800 879 3337

Tong Ren Herb Company
1190 N.E 125th Street, Suite 12
North Miami, Fla 33161
1 305 899 8704

Shen Nong Herbs
1600 Shattuck Ave
Berkeley, California 94709
1 510 849 0290

Bazaar of India
1810 University Ave
Berkeley California 94703
1 800 261 7662

Spring Wind Herbs
2325 Fourth St #6
Berkeley, CA 94710
1 510 849 1820

Monterey Bay Spice Company
241 Walker Street
Watsonville, CA 95076
1 800 500 6148 Fax: 722 3405

Acknowledgments

I want to mention my thanks to those who in one way or another contributed to this work coming to its conclusion.

Omar Martínez, editor, proofreader, and indispensable contributor, who has demonstrated an incomparable patience to correct the enormous barbarities that my limitations in the use of the computer have imposed.

Lester Triguero, who photographed most of the images in the book, got photos that were sent to him from Cuba, sent and received emails and helped me with the technology.

Dionnys Pino (mother of Lester Trigero), who kindly collaborated with the review of the testimonies.

Silvestre López (Pupi), who sent photos of plants from South Florida, USA.

Fermín Arias who got me photos of plants in the Dominican Republic through the collaboration of family and friends from different places in their country of origin.

Elito Cuellar, nephew of my wife Yolanda, sent me photos of plants from Cuba, in one of them, you can see the Cangrejo river, Fomento, Las Villas, Cuba, the freshwater beach of my youth.

Alberto Martínez junior, my beloved son who gave me the computer with which I started this work and another with which I finished, in addition to collaborating decisively in the edition of this book (thanks) and set up my website www.NJApitherapy.com .

Iker Arizmendi, my nephew, who gave me an iPad and a Laptop used in the creation of this book, and helped me with the technological problems that have never been missing.

Tanya Miranda, wife of my nephew Iker, auto-publisher of science fiction, fantasy and poetry, and computer programmer, helped me in translating, formatting and editing my book. Your help and patience was extraordinary! And also the sandwiches she offered me.

Maite Martinez, my dearest daughter, who also helped me with the logistical support without which this book could not have been finalized.

Yolanda, my wife from 50 years ago, who makes me happy with her presence alone, although she always asks me (with little result) to be more orderly.

And above all to God, who endowed me with enormous patience and willpower to always continue forward.

About the Author

The author is a passionate student and researcher of apitherapy and natural medicine. He is a retired professor of math and science who studied physics and mathematics at the University of Santa Clara, Cuba. His love for bees and the products of the beehive began more than five decades ago, in Cuba, his country of origin, where he was a beekeeper since his youth, and when for the first time he could appreciate the wonderful healing properties of the products of the bees.

Today, after thousands of hours of study and research, he says that apitherapy can produce very positive, and sometimes spectacular, results in the lives of people who dealt with other branches of medicine without obtaining the expected benefits.

Qualifications:

- Apitherapist: CAMC Exam "Charles Mraz" of the AAS
- Certified Herbalist: TCM, Western and Ayurveda Herbologist Consultant
- Digitopuncture (Acupressure): Tuina-Shiatsu. Based on TCM meridian theory.
- Naturopathy Doctor: Nutrition, Food Therapy, Minerals, Vitamins.
- Certificate in Chi Lel-Qi Gong: Breathing Exercises, Smooth Movements.
- Certification in Kinesiology - Touch for Health I-II
- Certification in Healing Reconnection - Reconnective Healing I-II

To learn more about the author, visit his website:

www.njapitherapy.com

Made in the USA
Middletown, DE
26 May 2023

30827892R00126